Breathe
to
Function

An Occupational Therapist's Guide
to Managing Shortness of Breath

Chris Kmiecik

Breathe
— to —
Function

An Occupational Therapist's Guide
to Managing Shortness of Breath

Chris Kmiecik

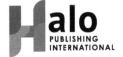

Halo
PUBLISHING
INTERNATIONAL

ISBN: 978-1-61244-907-4
LCCN: 2020918863

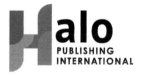

Halo Publishing International, LLC
8000 W Interstate 10, Suite 600
San Antonio, Texas 78230
www.halopublishing.com

Printed and bound in the United States

Acknowledgements

I would like to thank all of my co-workers and my family for their input and encouragement. Additionally, I need to thank, with all my heart, my niece and her husband, Ashley and Cory Austin, for their help with the book's editing process. And thank you to my dear wife, Connie, for all her help, guidance, and support.

Preface

If you or a loved one is having issues with shortness of breath and related fatigue, this book is written for you. My goal is to present you with the successful treatment strategies I developed in my practice as if I were in the room with you. Breathe to Function compiles what my coworkers and I have learned and utilized during our careers in various hospital settings and in homecare. Most of my career has revolved around the care of our patients, and their families, in their homes. If you were our patient, while under your doctor's care, we would provide education pertaining to your diagnosis, along with therapeutic treatment that would help you return to your prior level of functioning and independence. As your occupational therapist, I could use my collective training and beneficial patient experiences to guide you in the recovery from and the management of shortness of breath if needed, with the primary goal of helping you resume your daily activities. To gain your trust in my program and promote its benefits, I would learn your interests and goals, share some of my own, maintain a desire to succeed, and inject as much humor into the treatment as possible. Laughing will do as much as singing when it comes to getting you to breathe. You earn bonus points for either. As an occupational therapist, it is always thoroughly engaging to find out what is not working right...and to help fix it!

Contents

Disclaimer

Please use this book under the guidance and care of your physician. Your doctor will diagnose the cause of shortness of breath and related fatigue. Occupational therapists generally assess patients after they have received their medical evaluations from their physicians. The referral process is when the physicians call the rehabilitation teams (rehab) about patients who have been stabilized and are ready for rehab treatment. Basically, they are in "the medical system." If you are not in the medical system, or if you have not been medically screened, and you develop symptoms such as increased shortness of breath and fatigue during activities, please see your medical care provider for assessment and guidance. Early intervention is the key to maintaining good health and avoiding further injury.

The cardiovascular and pulmonary systems involve the heart and lungs, which are working to effectively meet the blood/oxygen needs of our bodies. Any disruptions in these areas can cause many symptoms, including shortness of breath and fatigue. That is why, prior to any medical procedure, there is an evaluation done by cardiologists and pulmonologists to ensure that our bodies can handle the stress of surgery and therapies. If you have not been seen by your doctor and you experience increased frequency in shortness of breath or fatigue, it is important that you notify your doctors and have yourself checked out. If you experience sudden shortness of breath or fatigue that is not related to an activity, seek immediate medical attention by calling 911.

Introduction

I have served in the profession of occupational therapy for thirty years. Over the last twenty years, I provided patient care as a homecare occupational therapist (OT) through the Cleveland Clinic Home Care department, from which I recently retired. Occupational therapy teaches our patients how to regain lost function following any life-altering event. The activities that "occupy" us during the day are called activities of daily living. The last time I checked, that would be just about everything! As an OT working in homecare, I had the opportunity to address health issues that might be restricting our patients' ability to function independently at home. The variety of daily activities that engage our patients at home required us to continually problem-solve and therapeutically instruct in normal or adaptive ways to help them regain any lost function. As a medical professional working on the front lines of patient care, I could not have chosen a more challenging and rewarding career.

Occupational therapy is a rehabilitation discipline. The OT is a member of a rehabilitation team that also includes physical therapy, speech therapy, nursing, social work, and respiratory therapy. In homecare, our functioning was supported by a bank of office staff, supervisors, schedulers, insurance precertification nurses, and our homecare aides. We all focused on the care and treatment of individuals who had limited ability to engage in or resume their daily functioning due to illness, injury, or developmental disability. Occupational therapists provide training that will help restore functioning for those folks with a medical condition that alters their ability to perform routine or daily activities. During rehabilitation or rehab training, our patients may present with breathing difficulties while engaging in activities of daily living. Effective breathing is one component of functioning that I highly focused on while providing treatment and education to meet their needs. I often found that when initially assessing a patient for the treatment of one medical condition, he or she may already have had a pre-existing breathing complication. For example, if the patient was recovering from hip surgery, it was during those early stages of recovery that we found that he may need some coaching on how to breathe more effectively. If someone already had a history of lung disease, his breathing could be further compromised, as well.

I had the opportunity to work as an OT at several hospitals during my career in Cleveland, Ohio. Early in my career, during the mid-90s, while working as a contract therapist, I was assigned to provide occupational therapy services to the patients at Grace Hospital, located in the Tremont area of Cleveland. It was a small neighborhood hospital. One of the hospital wards had been dedicated to supporting a new patient-care concept in what is now called a long-term, acute-care facility (LTAC). Basically, an LTAC is a type of hospital service that was developed to help care for extremely sick patients who required medical care and treatment for a long time. Some of those patients had complex pulmonary needs and were on ventilators continually, as they were unable to breathe on their own.

While at Grace Hospital, I had the opportunity to provide my OT services while learning how to treat breathing-compromised patients under a fine rehabilitation and respiratory therapy team. The medical director was the staff pulmonologist, and he guided the therapies directly. The hospital director had assembled a wonderful team. Everybody knew each other, and we worked well together. We were able to easily communicate daily with staff, families, and physicians. The staff worked closely together in order to implement patient care and advance treatments. Each week a team meeting was scheduled, and every discipline was in attendance, including the pharmacist. Pulmonary guidelines for ventilator-patient care were instructed, coordinated with rehab, and advanced by the medical director's team. Our rehab team's goal was to help get some of those extremely sick people off the ventilators and back to functioning individuals, which was a tall order.

The knowledge I gained while working with the Grace Hospital staff and respiratory therapy team guided my future occupational therapy treatment approach for managing patients with breathing difficulties. As an OT working for the Cleveland Clinic Home Care, I used what I had learned to address breathing difficulty with my patients in their own homes. It developed into a specialty area of interest and became a program that I taught my patients. I wanted my team to know that if there was a patient with a breathing issue, I wanted to know about it so I could help treat it. I have had success with my treatment program, and it has led to positive feedback reports from the patients, their families, and the rehab team.

As I am just recently retired and not actively treating, I wanted to share this treatment instruction in a written format so that patients, their families, and their caregivers could learn and apply it for themselves. I try to avoid the long-winded medical detail and provide you with a relevant, "hands-on" type of instruction, as if I were present and instructing with you there. A summary, or "cheat sheet," is provided at the end of this book. It includes the breathing exercises and safety considerations, along with page numbers, so you can easily reference the corresponding information located in this book. I would recommend reading the preliminary information prior to each exercise, as this will aid in the setup, understanding, and successful completion of each of the exercises. I will have videos on YouTube that you can access. They will provide visual reference to these breathing instructions. Please ask your doctor if you feel further guidance is needed. There are many well-trained therapists who can help you manage breathing difficulties.

In my experience as an occupational therapist, this is how I proceeded. During the initial assessment for occupational therapy, if the patient had a history of lung disease or became short of breath easily, I would start this breathing training program. This would have the patient learning how to manage shortness of breath at that moment. This helped me focus on what concerned the patient the most at that time. I would make this a part of his treatment plan and begin to instruct using this **breathe to function** program. Initially, the treatment was to ensure that the patient was using an effective breathing pattern. If the patient was able to understand and incorporate the "puffy cheeks breathing" technique that I instructed, I would usually see some of his anxiety diminish. It would take about fifteen minutes of instruction, and its focus was on an immediate need. This started the process and was the basis for the first exercise of a program designed to improve breathing performance. With practice, the patient was able to use this technique to help improve the effectiveness of each breath. This had a calming effect, which could then be used to help build confidence in managing his shortness of breath. The rest of this occupational therapy program would educate and provide training on how to breathe while improving endurance to perform and further engage in daily activities.

1

The Need to Breathe Effectively, Slow it Down and Relax Those Muscles

When you arrive at a hospital or medical clinic and present with shortness of breath, the medical staff assesses it quickly. They observe for symptoms, ask you what helps, and provide calming reassurance while administering their assessment protocols. The nurses instruct you on how to slow your breathing down and how to relax by using a technique called "pursed lips breathing." This technique has you breathe in through the nose and then form the lips to blow out of the mouth, like you're blowing through a straw. The nurses I knew had a saying to help you remember how to do this: "Smell the roses and blow out the candles." This activity is a quick way to show you how to ensure that your breathing is moving oxygen in and carbon dioxide out of the lungs. As your body becomes better oxygenated, it has a calming effect. This is a technique that has you focus on breathing in order to get that breathing to slow down and therefore breathe more effectively.

Let's learn how this technique works. While pursing the lips, the musculature of your mouth forms the lips in a tight, small circle or opening that helps resist the outward flowing air during an exhale. That resistance builds a little pressure, which helps to empty the lungs at that time. When this lip pursing is done, you look like you're going to give a kiss, like you're going to smooch with someone. That "smooching" position requires muscular effort to form those lips. A variation of pursed lips breathing that I instruct is called "puffy cheeks breathing." Puffy cheeks breathing is a technique that, in my opinion, works better. It has your lips relaxed during the exhale, and it feels more natural to use while performing an activity. The goal of both breathing techniques is to build up a little pressure in order to improve the effectiveness of the exhale. In practice, using the puffy cheeks technique takes advantage of the elasticity or "rubberiness" of your mouth to more easily and efficiently create that pressure during exhalation.

This breathe to function program also looks to improve upon the effectiveness of overall breathing by using less muscular effort and conserving energy. To breathe while using less muscular effort is the strategy I used to help most people troubled by shortness of breath during daily activities. The focus of this is to conserve your energy and to utilize the body's form and function in a way that is helpful to the breathing process. The breathing instructions presented here are appropriate for all levels of recovery. They can be utilized by the highly independent individual driving to the grocery store, just as they can be used by the person who requires assistance and is on bed restrictions or is bed-bound.

When a person exhibits shortness of breath with activity, there are many components that can potentially compromise the efficiency of his or her breathing. For example, perhaps he is breathing too quickly or panting. He may possibly be overusing the chest muscles and not relying on the diaphragm. He could have congestion or secretions in the lungs. Sometimes it is the way he is sitting; maybe he has poor posture. These things can limit how the air moves freely into our lungs. The muscles that support our bodies require oxygen to work. If we use "more" muscles to breathe, that activity uses up additional oxygen, which may further contribute to shortness of breath. If the overworking of those muscles is contributing to shortness of breath and creating more difficulty getting the breath back, it can lead to increased anxiety and stress, which will limit a person's desire to do things. That anxiety level and stress put the body in a heightened or tense state, which can also use up oxygen reserves in the blood. How can anyone relax with all of that going on? This is where it requires focus and planning in order to prevent yourself from moving into a heightened state.

Who could benefit from learning how to relax? Everybody! Deep breathing is a natural activity used by many disciplines for relaxation training. I often told my patients that the Chinese had invented deep breathing for relaxation a thousand years ago, and we stole it from them. In the present day, we find many benefits from using breathing to help us relax. Women are taught this for child birthing in Lamaze classes. It can also help to reduce anxiety and relieve pain, and it can help us to fall asleep. Deep breathing is also used as an exercise to expand the lungs.

Clinically, deep breathing is utilized as a pulmonary treatment or therapeutic exercise. It is how we are instructed to move larger amounts of air into our lungs. Patients are told to breathe in fully and to let it out slowly. This is a lung expansion exercise and is designed to increase lung volume and move air deeper into the lungs. This, too, has a calming effect and can be utilized to relax. Do this if you were instructed to do so by your pulmonologist or respiratory therapy team. Deep breathing, however, is not how we normally breathe with activity. Puffy cheeks breathing attempts to better ventilate the lungs during a typical respiration, without exaggerating the body movements while breathing. An efficient breath is the strategy we will use to relax ourselves. This is a more natural breathing pattern for learning how to breathe to function.

People who are diagnosed with a lung condition, or who experience shortness of breath with activity, benefit when they can get more of the "old air" out of their lungs while exhaling. Chronic obstructive pulmonary disease (COPD) is a slowly progressive lung disease that is characterized by lung function impairment with airway obstruction. Common symptoms are cough, sputum production, and shortness of breath (Ståhl et al. 2005, 56). COPD is the condition that typifies why I instruct this breathing strategy to manage shortness of breath. What happens with COPD is that during the process of breathing and upon the exhale, the airway obstruction tends to "trap" old air inside the lungs. As the person inhales again, he is moving fresh air in on top of the old air. A person with COPD has difficulty expelling all the old air so fresh, oxygenated air can get down deeper into the lungs. That is where the oxygen to blood transfer occurs. Over time, this diminished exhale develops into a poor pattern of breathing. The focus of this puffy cheeks breathing technique is not to emphasize getting the air in; it is to help those with lung function impairment get the bad air out! If that person can apply a more efficient exhaling strategy, the fresh air he then breathes in may find its way deeper into the lungs. This breathing strategy can work for most breathing conditions as well as for someone who simply becomes short of breath while overdoing it during an activity or exercise. For all breathing conditions, it is imperative to follow your doctor's instructions, manage and take all medications on time, and utilize prescribed oxygen appropriately.

Can we adapt our breathing patterns to meet our needs if we are getting short of breath during activities? Can we use this technique to relax? For my patients, I would encourage them by saying yes. It is not like taking another pill to relax; it is just relaxing by relearning how to make the breathing work for you. The goal of this book is to help you learn how to breathe with your normal body movements while becoming more efficient at exhaling. Effective breathing can help manage shortness of breath, build confidence, and avoid anxiety. If you can learn to relax better using these techniques, then build confidence in the performance of them, you can then work to improve your endurance with everyday activities.

As a therapist, I often see that breathing needs to be addressed for my patients during rehabilitation. There are many medical conditions that may compromise the breathing: COPD, asthma, pulmonary fibrosis, congestive heart failure (CHF), and pneumonia, to name a few. Perhaps we are just physically out of shape. What complicates matters is that, when diagnosed with a medical condition that affects the breathing, our activity levels may be curtailed. When we have difficulty engaging in our daily routines with vim and vigor, that medical condition can cause us to progressively weaken or decondition.

Deconditioning is a medical term used to define a progressing, intolerable weakness with ongoing related fatigue. When a person is weak from a previously described medical condition, he can become vulnerable to getting worse. As a therapist, I am called upon by the doctor to work with his patients in varying states of medical recovery. I will complete a chart review for the patients' relevant backgrounds and medical status information. I assess for functional limitation, develop a plan of care if needed, and then monitor the output and performance tolerance of those patients during some daily activity. I give them instruction on how to safely engage in exercise or activity and then monitor their progress. I can then adjust the intensity of that workout or activity over time to achieve a desired goal. If breathing or fatigue becomes difficult to manage when working toward a goal, it would be identified, and the plan of care would be adjusted to meet the patients' current activity level needs. It was my practice to identify any breathing difficulties while performing daily activities, assuring that the doctor was aware, and treating them accordingly. In most cases, breathing difficulties altered how my patients participated in their daily activities.

Lung conditions that challenge our breathing can be quite anxiety-provoking. I found that many patients would challenge themselves to engage in activities that would increase their shortness of breath. They would just try to "work through it" and push themselves. They would try to walk as far as they could while not stopping, for example, because they knew there would be a chair at the location they were headed to. Some would not stop walking due to the fear that they would become too short of breath and would have no place to rest at that moment. By the time they got to their destination, they were often so short of breath that they couldn't even talk. The "drive" to push through is admirable, but it is a self-defeating strategy, and it wears you down. This overworking is what pushes the blood oxygen level down in the body and makes it hard on a person to recover. My strategy was to learn breathing techniques and strategies that conserve energy. When practiced and applied, it has us working in manageable time frames while under control. This prepares us so that, when implemented, it can keep us more at ease. Becoming more at ease with our breathing can cure many ails.

When a person becomes short of breath, he can't think of anything other than getting that breath back. There cannot be anything more anxiety-producing than having difficulty breathing. How can someone remain active with such a challenge? I would often observe how people attempt to cope with this, and see an accelerated breathing pattern. In a state of rapid breathing and trying to deal with any mounting anxiety, there is a tendency to overwork the muscles in the upper body. It is an attempt to help "catch our breath." This accelerated breathing pattern is an example of compensatory breathing.

Compensatory breathing is how our bodies react and respond when a typical breath pattern does not feel adequate or does not relieve shortness of breath. Signs of compensatory breathing are open mouth breathing, panting, and exaggerated chest or upper body movements while breathing. One of the problems with this is that, with exaggerated chest breathing, it may neglect the use of the diaphragm, which is the primary muscle for breathing. For the most part, this breathing response is not efficient and can cause overworking of accessory muscles. Accessory muscles are the secondary muscles of the body, and they support our breathing. We are vulnerable to straining or overworking ourselves when we rely mostly on those muscles to breathe. When teaching my patients the breathing exercises and techniques, it required them to be in a calm state. We would then identify the activities that led to accelerated breathing. I would show them how to use this new puffy cheeks breathing technique, try to recruit the use of the diaphragm, and help them learn to breathe with their body movements in order to assist their breathing patterns. It may be difficult to identify a compensatory breathing pattern when a person's breathing is at rest, but it really shows itself when he is active or when the breathing becomes labored.

II

Breathing Exercises and Treatment Strategies to Improve Shortness of Breath

What Is Puffy Cheeks Breathing?

One of the most important concepts I wish to convey in this book is how to relax your breathing and make it more efficient by using a technique I call puffy cheeks breathing. As mentioned earlier, the technique that is taught by medical staff to slow your breathing if you are short of breath is pursed lips breathing. This technique uses the musculature of your lips and cheeks to form an opening of the mouth that slows the exhale. The formation of pursed lips makes us look like we are going to kiss someone or give a smooch. The muscles for smooching act to tighten the lips and cheeks. When doing this, those muscles use up oxygen while they are working. When you have shortness of breath and are trying to catch your breath, it makes sense to minimize additional muscular activity. In the first exercise, you will learn to relax the muscles of the mouth when exhaling by using puffy cheeks breathing. Note: For my cheat sheet users (pg. 113), I recommend reading this preliminary information to prepare yourself for each of these exercises.

1. Puffy Cheeks Breathing

This breathing program looks to improve upon the effectiveness of breathing by using less muscular effort. Breathing while using less muscular effort is the strategy I teach in order to help most people troubled by shortness of breath during daily activities. The purpose of this is to conserve our energy and use the body's form and function in a way that is helpful to the breathing process. The first example of this is how it applies to the muscles of the mouth when using the puffy cheeks breathing technique.

The use of puffy cheeks breathing is a technique I first learned of while co-treating with a respiratory therapy team. It was one of the breathing techniques they utilized to help improve their patient's' breathing. It was a strategy that I felt was easy to use during activities, and it seemed to be effective at improving breath performance. I found it to be helpful for myself in getting my breath back following the exertion during a heavier workout—after hiking up a steep hill, for example. If you watch the joggers, they are doing this thing with their lips when they run, and it helps them regulate their breathing. From these experiences, I wanted to ensure that effective breathing was a part of my occupational therapy training program. I would instruct on how to implement this breathing technique while treating my homecare patients, if they were experiencing any breathing difficulties that might be causing shortness of breath, fatigue, or anxiety-related issues.

The puffy cheeks breathing strategy relies little on the muscles of the mouth to exhale; instead it uses the flexibility or "rubberiness" of the lips and cheeks like a valve or a regulator. This characteristic of our mouths can be utilized to help restrict the flow of exhaled air coming out of our lungs. As the flow of air is restricted behind those relaxed, puffing lips and cheeks, it creates a "back pressure" during the exhale. This back pressure, called positive expiratory pressure (Olsen et al. 2015, 297-307), creates a gentle force that goes back down into the lungs and helps to hold the lungs open while you exhale. This action helps to get more of the bad air out so that, upon the next inhale, fresh air can move deeper into the lungs. A better exhale is what is so helpful for our patients with COPD, but it can also help most anyone having shortness of breath. This is a passive technique that assists the exhale. A passive technique is one that is using less muscular effort to perform. It teaches us how not to force the exhale or feel the need to "push the air" farther out of our lungs. Pushing is not necessary while using this breathing technique. Pushing the air out is a specific breathing strategy and should only be attempted if you are instructed to do so by your doctor or respiratory therapy team.

When exhaling with puffy cheeks in this manner, the cheeks puff out slightly, and you will hear the air pushing out through your relaxed lips. This technique uses the natural structures of the mouth to exhale more efficiently.

When learning this, you will blow out of the mouth with puffy cheeks and look like Marlon Brando's character in the movie The Godfather. They puffed out his cheeks with cotton balls to make him look mean. Along with this, the sound you will hear when blowing out with relaxed, puffy cheeks is the noise made while the air is being released. This is what builds up a little pressure behind the lips. It sounds like a flat tire going "pfffph."

Let us try it now. Breathe in through your nose gently and exhale through your mouth with puffy cheeks, comfortably, until you feel the need to breathe back in again. You will look like Marlon Brando and sound like a flat tire. If you are not sure you are doing it correctly, practice a few times and then go to a mirror and check to make sure your cheeks are puffing out and you are making a flat tire noise. If you start laughing or coughing, stop and try again later. Of course it will look funny at first, but with practice it will be much less noticeable. Coughing is a good sign. This exercise may loosen phlegm or congestion in your lungs. I know it sounds gross, but spit whatever comes out into a tissue, or swallow it. Do not allow it to get back into the lungs. Also, drinking enough fluids helps to keep the secretions moist and may improve your ability to have a productive cough.

A normal respiratory rate at rest is 12-20 breaths per minute (Cleveland Clinic 2019). A breath cycle is the time it takes for one inhale and one exhale. One breath cycle at rest normally takes about one second to breathe in and two to three seconds to breathe out. I call this our normal breath rate. This should feel like a comfortable rate of breathing. While performing my breathing exercises at rest, we are trying to stay close to these breath rates or ratios (the ratio is one to inhale and two to three to exhale). When performing puffy cheeks breathing, the cheeks act as the guide to keep your breathing within these time-frames. When you practice, breathe at the rate that feels comfortable to you. Once you feel comfortable breathing this way, the puffy cheeks breathing will maintain this ratio for you. You will not have to think about how long it takes to breathe. (See my YouTube video channel for puffy cheeks breathing [PCB] demonstration.)

While doing the breathing exercises, if you breathe too quickly, you may experience lightheadedness. Take a rest and then repeat a little slower after you ensure you are no longer lightheaded. If you breathe too slowly, it may not feel as if it is helping. The goals are to learn how to breathe this way and to make it match how fast your body is wanting to breathe comfortably. What if it's not comfortable because you don't normally breathe in through the nose?

If the nose is blocked or you are not a nose breather, then breathe in the mouth and exhale out of the mouth with puffy cheeks. There are many people who do not use their noses to breathe. They may have narrowing of the nasal passageways. Others have allergies or sinus congestion. I call them Cleveland noses. Due to the local allergies and inclement weather, at certain times of the year, it seems as if we all have runny or stuffed-up noses that don't seem to work right. Initially, I like to assess this by asking the patient, "How much air is moving into your nose when you inhale through the nose?" I would also ask, "When you breathe in your nose, how much air is flowing in freely? All of it, half of it, or less than that?" If I am told 50% or less, I would then ask my patients to breathe in using both the mouth and nose. Ensure that the amount of air moving in feels good. The air must move in freely!

Difficulty using the nose to breathe is a point that may sometimes be missed when medical staff instructs on the use of the pursed lips breathing technique to help people with shortness of breath. They will ask you to "breathe in your nose and then blow out your mouth, like blowing through a straw." However, if a person does not or cannot breathe in with the nose, he is less likely to use this breathing technique. Breathing strategies are important to help move air into and out of our lungs. If you are being asked by your doctor or nurse to breathe this way, there is most likely evidence that your breathing is inadequate at that time. For my instruction, whether it is breathing entirely in the mouth or the nose, it is most important that you exhale through your mouth when it is time to exhale. Let's learn how to use the lips to better resist an exhale with puffy cheeks.

If a person appears to have difficulty making puffy cheeks with their exhale, he may not be a good mouth breather. Verify this by having that person, or a helper, hold a tissue about six inches in front of his mouth and then have him practice blowing at the tissue to see it move. If the tissue moves freely as he blows, then it just takes practice to make the puffy cheeks. If it does not move freely, the patient is exhaling mostly through the nose.

For the person who can exhale out of the mouth but has difficulty with forming puffy cheeks, have him practice by making the "motorboat noise." That sounds like "making raspberries" with loose, floppy lips. Do you remember making that funny sound while blowing onto a baby's belly for giggles? I call it the motorboat noise. A big boat, with an inboard motor. It must be a loose-lipped sound like "flub, flub, flub." Not a small, outboard motor that sounds raspy, like "pssst." That sound means the lips are held tightly. Relax those lips and cheeks. (See YouTube video [PCB] for relaxed/tight lip breathing/nose breather exercise.) Practice making the motorboat noise for three sets of five repetitions, with 15 seconds of rest after each set. As those lips and cheeks relax, we will use this motorboat noise technique to improve the puffy cheeks breathing exercises. To review, this technique has the top lip resting gently on the lower lip. Now, blow or exhale through those relaxed lips. Avoid forming or opening the lips. Blowing through them in this way is what creates a little resistance, which helps to empty the lungs.

If you or your loved one has difficulty exhaling through the mouth, it may be that you are a nose breather. Practice by blowing at the tissue, using the mouth. As it becomes easier, increase the challenge by blowing at a pinwheel or heavier paper, such as a paper towel. Practice this as an exercise activity at the same frequency as the motorboat-noise exercise for a week or two. If better able to coordinate the mouth breathing, then try it with the puffy cheeks breathing exercise. Otherwise, continue using the pinwheel for this part of the breathing exercise. If shortness of breath with activity continues to present itself, ensure that the doctors are aware of this type of "nose breathing pattern." They may recommend respiratory therapy for additional breath training.

If you generally breathe in the mouth only, you are more likely to have mouth dryness. Having water nearby or at the bedside should help alleviate that dryness. While attempting to manage dry mouth, I recommend short sips to moisten. Try to avoid overdrinking for a dry mouth. Just a short sip of water to spritz and refresh your mouth should be effective. No need to guzzle and increase trips to the bathroom.

The next point about the use of the puffy cheeks breathing technique is that, when practiced regularly at rest, you become really good at it. It can help anyone who is in need of "catching his breath" to catch it more quickly. As your puffy cheeks technique improves, you will find that it is easier to breathe this way than using pursed lips breathing. It is a more natural use of the mouth and lips while you are moving about. As it tends to feel more natural to perform, you will be more inclined to use puffy cheeks breathing when you get short of breath. That is when it is most needed. I ask all my patients to perform their breathing exercises three times a day for each of the exercises instructed. The practice is what makes the breathing feel more natural. The exercises are relatively easy and can be practiced while seated at any time. The repetition of the exercises is what improves the puffy cheeks breathing technique. This technique is so important because it minimizes shallow breathing. To help motivate and encourage them to practice, I would tell my patients that I wanted them to become the best puffy cheeks breather in the neighborhood! Once you feel that it works, you can use it like a tool—a tool to help you breathe if you become short of breath.

Shallow breathing can occur when we get short of breath. This can lead to open mouth breathing or panting. Panting is good for puppy dogs but not for people who have breathing difficulties. This type of shallow breathing does not produce an efficient exhale and can be a poor pattern of breathing. Shallow breathing does not help us because it is not getting the fresh air deeper into the lungs. Puffy cheeks breathing creates that resistance to the exhale and helps prevent panting or shallow breathing. It helps to produce a full exhale.

The issue with panting or quick, open-mouth, shallow breathing is that it is not conducive to getting air deeper into our lungs. The windpipe branches of the lungs end at the alveolar sacs. The alveolar sacs are at the deepest part of the lungs. This is where the transfer of oxygen and carbon dioxide occurs, moving in and out of the blood stream, respectively. When we pant or shallow breathe, the air partially enters the lungs. The air is directed into the lungs by the trachea, brachia, and bronchioles; these are the windpipes. When we shallow breathe, the air is moved in and out of the lungs through these "pipes," but it may not be effectively reaching the alveolar sacs. Oxygen does not transfer into the bloodstream through the pipes. Therefore, panting or shallow breathing is not efficient. When short of breath, we really want to be efficient at breathing in order to get it back quickly.

When a person with normal breathing becomes short of breath following a vigorous activity, the respiration rate can increase to well over thirty breaths per minute. That means the breath rate goes faster, as well. Remember, while at rest, it normally takes about one second to breathe in and two to three seconds to breathe out. Even though he is breathing quickly, the normal breather maintains that one in to two-three out breath rate ratio (one split second in to two-three split seconds out). When you become short of breath, your breath rate changes. It gets faster. It may go to one split second to breathe in and one split second to breathe out. This breathing pattern, or ratio, (one in to one out) would have you panting. When breathing difficulties have been diagnosed, a shallow breath pattern may not sustain you. This can further lead to anxiety or prolong distressed breathing. To slow the breath rate, you will learn to add puffy cheeks breathing to the exhale. It supports the normal breathing ratio (one in to two-three out), which helps you avoid panting and improves breathing efficiency. Basically, this is what the nurses at the hospital are telling their short-of-breath patients. You relax by "slowing your breathing down."

For your training, while using this breathe to function program, it all starts with learning how to relax and better use the muscles that are the primary muscles for breathing. What about the muscles of the mouth? Instead of using the muscles to form your lips, as is done with pursed lips breathing, let's just relax them. You can use the soft suppleness of your lips and cheeks like a valve—a valve that resists that outward flow of air from your lungs during the exhale. This is the puffy cheeks breathing technique; it uses less muscular effort than pursing the lips. My goal is to help you learn this technique accurately as an exercise, and then you can use it to help your breathing should shortness of breath develop with activity. In all, there are three breathing exercises in this breathe to function program. They are the puffy cheeks breathing, ribcage breathing, and diaphragm breathing. The focus of these exercises is to learn the puffy cheeks breathing technique so that you can apply it to activity and then to improve upon muscular control, which helps your breathing.

1.- Puffy Cheeks Breathing / Exercise

Moisten your lips with your tongue. Rest the upper lip on the lower lip gently. Do not make an opening. Breathe in the nose gently with a small inhale, about one second. When ready to exhale, breathe out of the mouth through the relaxed lips with puffy cheeks, about two to three seconds. Exhaling with puffy cheeks should be comfortable and relaxed. Do not try to force more air out of the lungs at the end of the exhale, as this requires additional muscle activity. The puffy cheeks breathing helps to move the air out of the lungs for you. Practice breathing in and out using puffy cheeks. Do this five times; that is one set. Then rest for fifteen seconds. Repeat to complete three sets of five repetitions, and take a fifteen-second rest break after each set. Take your time and breathe easy. If you breathe too quickly, you may feel lightheaded. If lightheaded, rest and breathe easy. If breathing is fast, it can cause hyperventilation. It just takes some practice. When performed correctly, puffy cheeks breathing helps to prevent hyperventilation. It has a calming effect on the breathing.

Hyperventilation occurs when we breathe too quickly. This removes too much carbon dioxide from the body. Symptoms of this are lightheadedness, shortness of breath, belching, dry mouth, weakness or confusion, sleep disturbances, numbness and tingling in arms or around mouth, muscle spasms in hands and feet, and chest pain and palpitations (Hopkins Medicine). If you have any of these symptoms at rest and they persist or worsen, notify your physician, or seek medical attention. To learn how to monitor your breath rate, do it when rested. When taking yours or another person's respiratory rate, one inhale and one exhale is equal to one breath. To assess this, watch for chest rise and count the breaths using a clock with a second hand or a timer. An accurate assessment is when you take this for sixty seconds or take two thirty-second intervals and add them together. This reading will give you the number of breaths per minute and is called your respiratory rate. The normal respiratory rate is 12-20 breaths per minute at rest. Breathing at twenty-four to twenty-eight breaths per minute at rest is too fast. If you are breathing this fast, seek medical attention immediately. Conversely, if the breathing is less than twelve breaths per minute, this is too slow. If your doctor does not already know that the breath rate is this slow, seek immediate medical attention.

During the performance of puffy cheeks breathing, remember to breathe comfortably with your body. If you feel lightheaded because of the exercise, stop the exercise and breathe easy. Resume when this has cleared and slow your breathing pace during the exercise. You should only breathe as fast as your body needs to. Once you learn the technique and it feels comfortable, puffy cheeks breathing will slow the breath rate and, in turn, work to slow the breathing or respiratory rate. It can be quite relaxing.

To further review, the technique of puffy cheeks breathing, and the resistance that builds behind the closed, relaxed lips and cheeks, pushes the cheeks out slightly before the lips let the air escape when exhaling through your mouth. Because your lips are relaxed, it makes a soft hiss, like a flat tire sound. If you are having difficulty letting your lips relax—and many people do—try letting your lips flop as you exhale. That makes the bubbling noise like the motorboat engine while in the water at idle. "Blub, blub, blub." That is a good trick to get those lips to relax. As you get better at it, you will hear the flat tire sound or soft hissing. "Pfffph." Some folks just have tight mouths and lips, even at rest. Learn to relax them by pretending you're swirling mouthwash around your mouth with fat, puffy cheeks. That gets your cheeks going in the motion that is needed. For added visual feedback, try practicing this technique, and the exercise, while facing the mirror. I will post a video on YouTube that shows how to perform this technique. (See YouTube [PCB] "mouthwash" video.)

You are learning to use puffy cheeks breathing so that you can take action to help yourself should you become short of breath. When applying the puffy cheeks breathing, it will help to slow the pace of your breathing. In doing so, you do not have to think about how to breathe slower. The puffy cheeks breathing technique helps do this for you. It maintains the normal ratio even though you are breathing very quickly (one in and two to three out). The resistance created while blowing out the relaxed lips is what slows the exhale. It just takes a little more time for the air to push through the lips. The key to this is that the puffy cheeks are creating the needed resistance in the mouth which expels more of the bad air from the lungs upon exhale, especially when your breathing gets faster. At that point in time, it is a matter of implementing what you have learned. You will have to remind yourself to breathe this way if you become short of breath. It may look funny while you are doing it, because you are doing it so fast. But that is how fast your body is asking you to breathe at that time. If someone asks you what is it that you are doing, tell them you are doing your breathing exercise and that you will be right with them, or give them that "be right with you" sign. Repeat this puffy cheeks breathing pattern until the breathing relaxes. This is how you get your body to slow the breathing and avoid shallow breathing.

The practicality of this is that if you become short of breath, you are not saying, "Oh my gosh, I'm short of breath. What can I do?" I need you to think, "Oh! Chris said to do that puffy cheeks breathing." And breathe this way. That is why I want you to become the best puffy cheeks breather in the neighborhood. With practice, it will become like second nature, and like a tool, you will pull it out of your pocket and use it when needed. I would later quiz my patients and ask, "When breathing with puffy cheeks, which should take longer? Breathing in or out?" Answer: Breathing out.

Having you follow this exercise instruction from a book may be more difficult than if I were demonstrating it while standing in front of you. (See fast PCB video on

YouTube.) Just know that initially learning these exercises may not be as easy as it sounds. Many of my patients have had difficulty at first. Also, poor breathing habits can be hard to break. This puffy cheeks breathing technique is a relaxed exhale and is key to relaxing your overall breathing by improving exhale efficiency. It takes practice, but it's worth it! Once you master this, it becomes like a tool you can rely on to help get your breath back. When teaching the entire breathing program to my patients, it would take, on average, a part of two to three forty-five minute treatment sessions to learn the exercises and breathing programs, along with an additional two treatments to apply these instructed breathing techniques and energy conservation strategies to daily activities. Remember, for this first exercise, breathe in your nose gently and blow out the mouth with puffy cheeks. It makes you look like Marlon Brando, and you'll sound like a flat tire. As you practice this and your technique improves, the "look" and "sound" become much less obvious. Practice this when you are relaxed and take your time. As your technique improves, you will later learn how to add the puffy cheeks breathing if your breathing gets faster during more strenuous activity. The next exercise begins to show the impact of breathing with the rib cage.

2. Rib cage breathing using the upper body

The key to this next exercise again reinforces the fact that when we overuse muscles, they use up more oxygen. When a person is trying to get his breath back, it makes sense to minimize additional muscle activity. When patients have breathing difficulties, become anxious, or develop shortness of breath, the therapists see all kinds of extra muscle use and movement patterns. I referred to this previously as compensatory breathing. They are moving this way to help get their breathing under control. They are over relying on accessory muscles. Accessory muscles are the secondary muscles that support our breathing. Secondary muscles for breathing are found in the upper body, chest, back, neck, and upper arms. When over relying on these muscles for breathing, the chest and upper body start to overwork and become tense. To minimize that overworking tension at the chest and upper body, and to better use the accessory muscles, we can instruct in the use of upper body, chest, and rib exercises. Because of the anatomy of our rib cage, we can move the rib cage and exercise some of those accessory muscles with a simple exercise.

The ribs are connected in the back to the thoracic part of the spine or upper back. When we straighten our spine in this area, we are extending at the thoracic spine. We can make the rib cage rise by straightening the spine in our chest area. This can be done by sitting tall and raising the arms overhead. When the rib cage rises, it opens the lung space within and allows air to more easily move into the lungs. Let's do this as an exercise called the rib cage breathing exercise.

2.- Rib Cage Breathing / Exercise

Sit in a comfortable chair to learn this exercise. Push your hips back into the seat and sit up straight. If the chair is large, use a pillow in the lower back area. You will need this support. If you are able to move both arms overhead without pain, raise both arms overhead and feel the upper back (thoracic spine) straighten. It feels as though you are sticking out your chest. This movement will open the rib cage area and allow the lungs to expand. This movement helps us to inhale. When you lower both arms back down to the sides, the spine flexes, and the ribs return to their starting position. This direction moves the ribs downward, and it compresses the lung space. This movement can help you to exhale. Please do not attempt moving arms overhead if having pain or difficulty moving in this way. We can modify this exercise by straightening at the spine, without raising the arms. The rib cage breathing exercise combines upper body and chest movement with the puffy cheeks breathing. Let's do this. Breathe in through the nose while raising the arms overhead, about one second, and then blow out puffy cheeks while moving the arms down to your sides (takes about two to three seconds). Try to move the arms as fast as you are breathing while using this breath rate. Do this five times and then rest fifteen seconds after each set. Complete three sets of five repetitions.

Many of our patients are not able to raise their arms overhead without pain, as many have shoulder joint limitations. To accommodate painful shoulders, I can modify this exercise so you don't have to reach overhead. While seated in the same starting position, you will sit up straight while keeping your hands at your sides. Next, straighten at the back and stick your chest out while breathing in. The rib cage will rise while you're breathing in for about one second. Then, relax your upper back. The rib cage will lower as you blow out using puffy cheeks; this takes about two to three seconds. Do three sets of five repetitions, with a fifteen-second rest break after each set. Verify that you are not becoming lightheaded or having upper body pain. If lightheaded, discontinue this exercise and continue using the puffy cheeks breathing. You may be breathing too quickly. Breathe easy until it passes. If having pain, reduce the amount of back straightening and verify that you are not using your arms You may want to ask a helper to watch you for accuracy or to see if you are tensing up. If only one arm has discomfort with movement, you can raise the other arm with this exercise. The timing of this exercise, moving arms up and then down, should coincide with the breath rate. It is okay to breathe more times during the movement if you feel the need to do so. Just time the inhale to occur when arms or ribcage move up, and exhale when they come down. If pain is persistent or worsens with the breathing exercises, please notify your physician. It is possible that an injury that may not have been identified is lurking. A rib cage injury (ex: a rib fracture) that is undiagnosed may be the culprit that leads to complications. The next exercise looks to see how well the diaphragm muscle is contributing to your breathing.

3. Diaphragm Breathing

The diaphragm muscle is the number one muscle for breathing. It is located near the bottom of the rib cage, below the lungs and above the stomach. It is a relatively flat muscle that, upon inhale, works to pull downward on the space below the lungs, which then draws air into the lungs. This muscle relaxes when we exhale and then moves back up into position below the lungs. When we are born, for the most part, we all have normal, functioning diaphragms. It is as we get older when we can develop poor breathing habits and strategies that can lead to weakening of this muscle. Changes to our breathing patterns may occur as we age or when we experience difficulties in normal breathing. In response to this, we sometimes change our normal breathing patterns to an alternate breathing pattern that feels helpful. These alternate patterns are again called compensatory breathing patterns. To overcome breathing weakness or shortness of breath, many people learn to over rely on or "compensate" using other muscles. Those other muscles help or support breathing but are not meant to be the primary muscles for breathing. Those muscles are called the accessory muscles, and they use up much more oxygen when used as if they were the primary muscles for breathing. That is when we will see the overuse of the upper body and chest musculature. In addition, when a person is over reliant on chest musculature for breathing, we often see a lack of diaphragm use. As the diaphragm is the primary muscle for breathing, not using it can make it weaker. That can make our breathing less effective. Either the increased use of accessory muscles or lack of diaphragm control can lead to an increased reliance on compensatory breathing. These people are called "the chest breathers."

When people develop bad patterns of breathing, over time it becomes the "new" normal. To them it feels natural. A normal inhale should start from the diaphragm, at the belly. The tummy should start to expand just before the chest begins to rise. The chest breathers, on the other hand, pull air into the lungs using the upper body and chest muscles. They have learned to breathe mostly with their chests. When they inhale, the chest rises first. To complicate matters, society has taught that proper etiquette for women is to tighten their tummies and breathe with their chests. In my practice, I've found that women are more often the chest breathers. It must be a vanity thing. Men, on the other hand, are used to those beer bellies. They just let it all hang out. Men are generally good belly breathers. Remember, the diaphragm is the number one muscle for breathing. When it's working, the tummy should move outward when breathing in. Being a muscle, it can be strengthened or recruited into the "belly" component of breathing. We will learn the diaphragm exercise if you are more of a chest breather.

To find out if you use your diaphragm when you breathe, sit back and relax. Sit back in that recliner or lie on your back, positioned comfortably, in bed. This is a good position to see if you use your diaphragm, or a helper can observe the tummy while you breathe. The patient is asked to take three comfortable deep breaths. If you are assessing yourself, place one hand on your tummy at or above the navel, and place the other on the chest. A helper can also watch for tummy rise. The patient will feel how the tummy rises compared to the chest while three deep breaths are taken. If the tummy rises first and then the chest, this demonstrates good use of the diaphragm. If the tummy raises a little and the chest moves more, or if only the chest moves, the diaphragm is not being utilized effectively while breathing. We will need to wake up those tummy muscles. As the diaphragm is the number one muscle for breathing, we can exercise it in hopes of improving diaphragmatic control, which will aid the breathing process.

Preparation for the diaphragm breathing exercise:

The reclined position, or lying in bed on your back, is the best position to monitor or learn diaphragmatic breathing. Let's reintroduce you to the movements of the diaphragm and what it should look like. Can you recall or visualize Mom or Dad lying on their backs, the baby sitting on their tummies, giving the child the up/down ride? Dad would poke his tummy out, and with giggles, the baby would go up and down with the contractions of his stomach. This activity would engage his abdominal muscles and simulate the movement required in this exercise. Promoting abdominal control can engage the diaphragm muscle. For our chest breathers, this activity can "reawaken" the diaphragm using the abdominal muscles. This may be challenging. The chest breathers make little use of the abdominals and, most likely, the diaphragm when they inhale. Therefore, getting comfortable using the abdominal muscles is the first part of this exercise.

While comfortably reclined or lying in bed, place one hand on your tummy, just above the naval. Always keep your hand on your tummy, as you will feel for tummy rise. The other hand can be relaxed at your side. Try to push your belly button outward toward the ceiling using your tummy muscles. You should see and feel your hand moved outward by your belly. Poke your tummy out about an inch or two, then relax it and let the tummy go comfortably back to where it was. Try not to pull your tummy inward, as this works more muscles. Do three sets of five repetitions, with a fifteen-second rest break after each set. If the tummy just barely moves outward, consider it a success.

Sense what that movement feels like and be sure to repeat it during this exercise. If you do not feel any movement outward, you will need to work on those tummy muscles. Depending upon how difficult this is to perform, you may need to practice this task alone as the first part of the diaphragm breathing exercise. Just give this a good effort. Some people may have medical conditions that limit their diaphragm movement. Practice this belly-poking exercise for several days, until you can effectively complete it or you develop a sense that something is happening down there. When you can use your tummy muscles, you will add this movement to the breathing part of this exercise.

3.- Diaphragm Breathing / Exercise

Here is how I instruct a patient to breathe with this exercise. I would ask you to get into that comfortable, reclined position, with one hand on your belly. I would then ask you to practice by poking the tummy out and relaxing the tummy three times, ensuring that you feel the tummy moving up and down. On the third attempt to poke the tummy out, I would then tell you to breathe in at that exact time, then exhale and relax the tummy. Do not try to pull the tummy in during the exhale, as if trying to "push" more air out of the lungs. Again, that extra muscle movement uses up more oxygen. Just let the tummy relax as you exhale, and the belly will fall to its relaxed position. The key point here is learning to inhale at the moment you poke the tummy out. As this becomes easier, remember to "add" the puffy cheeks breathing to the exhale during this exercise. The gentle pressure that is created with puffy cheeks is what will push more air out of the lungs. Performing the puffy cheeks breathing with each of these exercises reinforces learning this technique accurately. It will help you to remember and reinforce the use of this technique when you need to manage shortness of breath with other activities. To review this exercise, place one hand on your tummy. Poke your tummy out and, at the same time, breathe in the nose for one second. Then exhale and relax your tummy while blowing out with puffy cheeks, about two to three seconds. Do three sets of five repetitions, with a fifteen-second rest break after each set.

The diaphragm muscle exercise may be the most difficult of these three exercises to coordinate. Finding your "abdominals," or tummy muscles, and engaging them may be harder than expected and will take some practice. Timing the inhale to occur at that instant also takes some practice. Bad breathing habits are also often hard to break. When people are chest breathers, they have neglected using their diaphragm and tummy muscles for a long time. They feel comfortable with chest breathing. It often only becomes an issue when they develop shortness of breath with activities or when experiencing another medical issue.

So, when this OT guy would come along and identify that chest breathing is a contributor to shortness of breath, I would simply tell my patient that they are breathing "backwards." During a normal breath, upon inhalation, the tummy should start to move outward, followed by chest expansion. When these patients breathe, the chest goes out first, with little or no outward movement of the tummy. The reality of what happens is that, when a chest breather inhales, his tummy actually goes inward. I would quiz my patients about the movements of the tummy when using their diaphragm while breathing. "When you breathe in, which way should your tummy go? In or out?" Answer: out.

The lack of diaphragm use is a huge indicator for why a patient can have shortness of breath. Good news! The diaphragm is a muscle. Provided that there is no injury to this muscle, and when exercised regularly, it can be strengthened. When good technique is learned, these three breathing exercises are easy and can be completed at any time. I ask my folks to do these at least three times a day. Initially, you can learn these while reclined in a chair or while lying with pillows for support on your back. Once you feel comfortable with your understanding of the technique, you can do these while seated upright in any chair. These exercises will become easy to practice and can be completed in under ten minutes. You can literally do these while watching television. Finally, I cannot overemphasize the importance of learning how to perform and practice these exercises accurately.

The breathing exercises will help make these muscles more responsive and aid in the breathing process. Once you have learned these exercises, a better position to do them is while seated upright. Do the exercises while sitting tall, with hips forward in a chair, so that your back is off the back cushion. This will straighten the spine and will help you find that comfortable position that allows the ribcage movement while exercising. Sitting upright and tall is an important and more advanced way to strengthen the postural muscles of the spine, which also support the breathing.

It is important to learn how to position our bodies to promote good breathing results. A comfortable, supported position makes it easier to breathe when you are relaxing or when performing these breathing exercises. The preferred position for initially learning these exercises is while seated back in a recliner or while on your back while supported in bed. Lying flat on the back in bed may not be tolerated well. Address this by using pillows to support the upper body and head on a slight incline. Avoid too much pillow under the head, as this over flexes you at the neck. A larger bed pillow positioned under both thighs and pulled close to your butt will rest the weight of your legs and flex you at the hips. This is the "hospital bed" position, with the head and knees elevated. This is a comfortable position for breathing while on the back, as it slightly flexes the spine and relaxes the rib cage area. When lying flat on the back, the thoracic part of the spine, or rib cage area, holds the rib cage elevated. That makes it feel like you are "pinned" back and restricts the rib cage movement that is needed for breathing. This is one reason why so many patients prefer to sleep on their sides. If you find comfort on your back in the hospital bed position, consider obtaining an adjustable bed.

If you are feeling weak or are having difficulty breathing while lying in bed, reclining in a recliner chair can be more comfortable. Do remember, though, that most recliner chairs and couches are too big for us. If your hips do not scoot back into the seat easily, it will flex you at the thoracic spine. It can be difficult to breathe when the spine is flexed at the ribs. An oversized chair will make you look like you are sitting in a teacup. Fix an oversized chair by placing one or two large bed pillows behind the back. A reasonably supported posture in sitting is important, as it allows us to breathe easier. Recliner chairs are also notorious for not providing enough lumbar support. Ensure that the pillow fits the low, curved part of the back, called the lumbar area. Otherwise, consider ordering a chair or recliner chair that is sized to the individual who will be using it. When ordering a chair, two important measurements to consider are: 1. Seat depth, measured from back of knees to back of the butt while seated upright; and 2. The width at the person's hips. Look online to determine all the chair measurements, or visit a trusted furniture store. It is important to know the user's measurements before purchasing.

Other options for positioning to improve breathing include side lying in bed or sitting. When side lying, place an oversized pillow or a large teddy bear in front of you so you can rest the top arm. It will look like you are hugging it. Don't squeeze him. You're only resting the weight of your arm on it instead of on your chest. When using a properly sized chair, use a small pillow at the lower back to ensure lumbar support. Consider an armchair that will give support to both arms. For couches or oversized chairs, consider using rolled or folded towels and padded boxes just under the elbows to support the weight of the arms; do this along with the back-support pillows.

If breathing is heavy following an activity, take a seat and then slightly lean forward and rest your hands on your knees. If a table is nearby, try sitting with arms folded on top. If needed, rest your head on your arms. Placing your arms on a surface in front of you helps to support the weight of your arms and upper body, preventing them from pulling down on your chest. Resting forward this way holds the spine and rib cage in a neutral position and helps to open the airways. Perform the puffy cheeks breathing as fast as you are breathing at that time, and this will help you catch your breath.

If the symptoms of increased shortness of breath persist or worsen, notify your physician. Verify that the doctors are aware of your condition and report any new signs or symptoms. Shortness of breath can come from other causes. For example, congestive heart failure (CHF), when active, may cause fluid build-up. The fluid can collect in the space around our lungs and other areas of the body. This can cause shortness of breath. If you were diagnosed with this condition, your doctor would have asked you to monitor your weight daily and to write it down. The daily weights can then be tracked and compared while looking for a weight gain or loss within a twenty-four-hour time span. They will let you know how much weight gain or loss should be reported. If it exceeds this, it is to be reported to the physician after taking the weights that morning. Always remember to perform puffy cheeks breathing with any shortness of breath. If you know you can relax yourself using these breathing techniques, you can better manage anxiety if you become stressed.

Taking medication on time, using prescribed oxygen, and taking aerosol treatments per instructed scheduling are important treatments prescribed to minimize shortness of breath. Strive to use these medications on time! The doctor is most likely aware of your situation and has provided you with the appropriate medications to manage your breathing symptoms. Aerosol treatments are more effective to stave off shortness of breath when taken on time or just before you need it. This manages the congestion that forms in the lungs daily. Ensure that you take them at those times of day, when you have difficulty managing congestion, and when you anticipate a stressful task. If need be, ask family or helpers to arrange reminder strategies to help you stay on schedule. For example, use a timer for the next aerosol treatment. Taking the medications on time and per dosing instruction is probably the most important strategy in your arsenal to manage symptoms of shortness of breath. Now, how can we learn to better manage shortness of breath with activities?

As a therapist, when helping my patients learn to manage shortness of breath and continue to function, my job was to set up a program that fosters independence and success. Oftentimes, the easiest way goes a long way. I found this learning concept was a good way to engage patients and, hopefully, recruit their active involvement in following through with the exercises and techniques. When a person is weak and trying to cope with breathing difficulties and they are confronted with a new or ongoing medical condition, they may become disheartened and lack enthusiasm to participate in exercise programs. This is why, upon our first meeting, I would always start my breathing training with one goal: to have my patient learn the benefits of puffy cheeks breathing. The use of this relatively simple technique gets people moving air in and out of their lungs. My empathy goes out to a patient with anxiety-related breathing difficulties. Anytime we can do better at getting oxygen into our blood, it has a calming effect. When my patients learned that their new breathing technique helped them to breathe, it was a good first step to helping them feel more comfortable, and I then usually had a captivated audience. If not eager, they were always at least interested in learning the next exercise, breathing strategy, or technique to help manage their shortness of breath. With that success, it prepared them to actively learn the remainder of this breathing program. What other things are needed to help us succeed? We cannot lose sight of basic everyday needs.

It's not difficult to understand how the little things in our lives can get missed when we are ill or feeling down. Ask yourself:

- Am I drinking and eating enough?

- Do I get enough rest and activity?

- Am I taking all my medications accurately and on time?

- Did I reschedule a follow-up visit with my physician?

- Do I use my oxygen correctly and maintain the equipment?

- What else could affect my breathing: dust, perfumes, allergies?

- Allergies to dogs, cats, or birds?

- Do I need extra help to keep up with things or assistance with getting them done?

For someone who has been ill and gets short of breath with activity, managing all his own cares on time can also become quite anxiety-producing. Anxiety alone can lead to shortness of breath. Please communicate with your family or physician if your daily chores or responsibilities feel overwhelming. Try to figure out the best way to get some help. Once you realize help may be needed, get this process going. If available to you, use your medical social worker (MSW). Each hospital or medical facility provides access to a social worker who will assist with discharge planning. Your doctor can order their services when you ask. These folks are truly knowledgeable and can instruct in most areas of stay-at-home needs and the services available to you in your community. In homecare, the social workers can provide valuable information and assistance to meet most people's needs. Whether the patient was functioning at a high level and had questions regarding finances or how to afford medications, or whether the patient had greater needs and required additional services to augment the family and helpers' care at his home, our social workers were instrumental in helping the homecare team manage that transition from the hospital, and they addressed any patient and caregivers needs in the home. It was the therapists' job to instruct and train the patient to safely perform his daily activities.

III

Learning to Breathe with Your Body Movements and Daily Activities

Do you experience shortness of breath or fatigue when getting dressed or when bathing? Some people get winded walking out to the mailbox. It is important to recognize when the breathing limits any daily activity. Therapists are trained to teach patients how to manage their recovery process and address any limitations. The occupational therapist helps by assessing whether a patient can complete his daily activities, like getting dressed, for example. Can that person complete a routine task like putting socks on? Some folks cannot reach their feet, some have surgical restrictions to follow, and some get short of breath when bending to reach their feet. Most people wish to regain their independence and resume their daily activities following an injury or a medical procedure. OTs can train patients on how to overcome their limitations, how to adapt to meet their needs and become more independent, or just how to make it easier. If shortness of breath or fatigue limits the ability to complete a task, we can instruct in a treatment strategy called energy conservation.

The energy conservation treatment is just what it sounds like, and it asks, Are you running out of energy because of your breathing or fatigue? If yes, then how do you conserve what energy you have, make it last, or, better yet, get some more! Energy conservation is how we alter our activities or change our surroundings to accommodate our fatigue levels. The therapist helps the patient to ask, "How can I conserve my energy so I can do what I choose to do without wearing myself out?" One part of energy conservation is learning to breathe effectively with how you move. I call it breathing with your body mechanics. It uses your body movements to help push the air out of or draw the air back into the lungs while you move. Whenever you move, there is a beneficial way to breathe during that movement based on the positioning of the rib cage. Recall exercise #2 on page 43. You learned when to breathe in or out with the arm movements. When the arms go up, the thoracic spine straightens and raises the rib cage, and that is when you should breathe in. When the arms go down, the spine flexes, and the rib cage lowers. That is when you should breathe out. If you become short of breath, use the puffy cheeks breathing to exhale. It's just a way to breathe as you go. If the breathing techniques assure us of one thing, it is that you are not holding your breath as you move. That is especially important!

Now let's apply the breathing with body mechanics techniques. When reaching overhead—into the kitchen cabinet, for example—you would breathe in as the arm goes up or away from your body. While lowering your arm back down to the counter, that movement makes it easier to breathe out. When you bend over at the waist, as if to reach under the sink, the spine flexes, and the rib cage compresses the lung space farther. You would then breathe out using puffy cheeks. When you return to standing, the spine straightens, and the rib cage expands; this is the time to breathe in. In addition, using puffy cheeks breathing while bending over at the hips helps us in another way. The slower exhale takes advantage of the stability the lungs can provide when they are full of air.

When the lungs are full, they exert an outward force on the rib cage, chest, and upper back. That force provides a stable support to this area of the body from within. Having the lungs full of air when we do something makes us feel stronger when we move the arms or bend over. Because of this, many people will hold their breath while exercising. It makes the movement feel easier. The problem is that when they rely on this breath-holding technique with exertion, it can build up too much pressure within the body. The therapists are always reminding their patients not to hold their breath during exercise for this reason. We can learn to better take advantage of the stability a full-lung rib cage offers by letting the air out slowly when moving or bending. Puffy cheeks breathing helps us to do this.

Releasing the air with puffy cheeks when bending at the hips while standing provides a mechanical advantage that can make you feel stronger with this movement. As always, try to breathe with how fast your body is telling you to breathe. Stop periodically to check for shortness of breath or fatigue. Take a rest as needed. It is the puffy cheeks breathing that acts to slow the respiratory rate if the activity causes you to breathe too quickly. Remember, you are learning to exhale more efficiently using puffy cheeks breathing and then incorporating the breathing into your body mechanics while moving about. These techniques will help you to conserve energy and ensure good breathing practice while you engage in an activity.

The next energy conservation strategy requires you to put on your thinking cap. It requires you to plan and prepare. If you have a breathing condition, you may get short of breath while dressing. Planning ahead helps to prepare your area and make it conducive for dressing. To conserve your energy, prior to dressing, you should move all clothing items and supplies near the place you get dressed, or have someone help you to set this up. This will save energy, as you will avoid the need to get up to retrieve items during this task. Sitting on a supportive armchair with clothing and supplies within reach uses less energy. Let's use these strategies to get dressed.

Now, let us learn how breathing with your body movements during a dressing task will conserve energy. When you put a shirt on, the arms will be moving overhead or away from your body. To use breathing with body mechanics, when your arm goes up or out as you poke an arm into the sleeve, you should breathe in. When the arm moves back down, you should then breathe out. If breathing becomes heavier when you are repositioning the shirt, use your puffy cheeks breathing during the task. If you are short of breath after pulling the shirt on, take a short break to help get your breath back. Always check for shortness of breath at intervals to prevent it from getting away from you. The sooner you start a rest break, the quicker you can recover. If rest breaks take longer or you have increased difficulty with recovery from any activities, let your doctor know. This is a good way to monitor your performance and bring awareness to any potential health difficulties. Now, let's get the pants on.

As you have learned, you can coordinate breathing with your body movements while reaching overhead or with upper body activities. While seated for the lower body dressing, coordinate the breathing by blowing out puffy cheeks as you bend over. While bending, the spine is flexing around the rib cage. This movement pushes the air out of your lungs. As you sit back up, breathe in through the nose. Now, add this breathing technique to the task of putting on pants. While holding the waistband of your pants, bend over to place it over your foot while blowing out. As you push your leg through and pull the waistband up, breathe in while sitting back upright. Repeat this pattern of breathing when bending and sitting back up for the other leg. Try to avoid holding your breath and breathe while you move. Breathe in as you move to standing so you can pull the pants up and position them over your hips. Blow out puffy cheeks when you go to sit back down. I will later discuss how it helps to coordinate your breathing when moving from sitting to standing (See page 85).

Socks can be the most challenging when dressing ourselves. When putting socks on, it may require additional time to position the sock over your foot. Most of us are usually inclined to stay bent over at the hips until that sock is on. I would recommend that you break this sometimes-difficult task into smaller pieces so that you can "come up for air." For example, with sock in hand, bend over while blowing out slowly with puffy cheeks. Position the sock over your toes and then sit back up while breathing in. Repeat this breathing and bending as you reach to move the sock a bit farther up and then onto your foot. If these tasks take longer than a normal breath, just breathe while working. Try to avoid staying flexed over at the hips or holding your breath. When you bend over and stay there, you are blocking your diaphragm from moving. This puts a strain on your body and may increase shortness of breath. For people who have greater difficulty bending over to reach their feet, try placing your foot on a footstool or, if no medical restrictions, crossing the legs to improve your reach. Sometimes it helps to use a tool like a sock starter to put the sock on (Health Products For You), or use a dressing stick to push the sock off or reposition it around the ankle (CWI Medical). This can reduce the strain of bending at the hips while putting those socks on. This is the one dressing task that, if too difficult, I recommend you ask for assistance or further training. When those tight support stockings are required, just ask for help. Now that you're dressed, let's go into the kitchen and help out. Before you go, though, let's talk.

There is an awful lot of breathing strategizing going on here. Leave it to a therapist to analyze every "body moving" component when you're trying to do things. The body movement and efficiency scientists love to hear all the intricacies of how to breathe effectively when they put their pants on. For many folks, on the other hand, they are just not into all that "analyzing." I would just ask them to breathe during the activities, avoid holding their breath, and take rest breaks as needed. I do, however, highly recommend puffy cheeks breathing, if you could not already tell. If you are more of the efficiency-expert type, then these breathing with body mechanics strategies, when implemented correctly, are effective to help conserve your energy.

When it comes to working in the kitchen, there are many ways the body moves. Here, you can take advantage of breathing with your body and conserve energy with most kitchen activities. Let's say that your helper went shopping and left the groceries on the counter. She bought spices, dish soap, and pot scrubbers. The spice rack is on the first shelf above the sink, and the cleaning supplies go under the sink. As you may still be weak from a given medical condition or procedure, set yourself up and work in the kitchen safely. First, turn a chair out from the table so that you can easily sit to take a rest break. When standing at the sink, always hold the counter with one hand, especially when reaching. As you are ready to reach overhead to put the spices away, face the cabinets and hold the counter with one hand and then open the upper cabinet door while breathing in. Bring the same hand down to grab the cinnamon while blowing out with puffy cheeks. Place the cinnamon on the first shelf while inhaling and then bring that hand down and exhale with puffy cheeks. Repeat the same steps for the thyme, rosemary, and sage. Stop here and check yourself. See if you are having any shortness of breath or fatigue. Consider a rest break if needed. Otherwise, perform puffy cheeks breathing while standing to catch your breath. If you feel no fatigue or shortness of breath, continue with putting the remaining spices away.

Next, the cleaning supplies go under the sink, so let's use the breathing while bending technique. Plan ahead and place the supplies on the counter, near the cabinet door beneath the sink. Turn yourself perpendicular to the sink so that you are facing down the length of the counter. In this position, your one hand rests easily on the counter. While holding the counter, exhale with puffy cheeks and bend at the hips and knees to open the lower cabinet door with your other hand. Breathe back in as you stand back up. With that same hand, grasp the dish soap. Now, as you bend over, blow out puffy cheeks and place the soap in that lower cabinet. Return to standing while breathing in (it helps if you hold onto the counter when standing perpendicular or sideways while bending over; it's easier and offers good support). Check to see if you are fatigued, short of breath, or lightheaded If so, move to the table and rest at that chair for a short time. Otherwise, repeat the same steps for putting the pot scrubbers away. See if this activity is enough for now.

Essentially, these are energy conservation techniques that have you breathing with your body movements. When you repeatedly engage in self-care and kitchen activities while adding these conservation strategies, it will teach you to breathe as you're working, offer guidance to improve your endurance, and, eventually, make you feel stronger and more confident. Basically, it is learning to breathe with your natural body movements.

Our bodies and ribs are natural air movers. If you were to ask a singer or a wind instrument musician, they know that our ribs and diaphragms are like the bellows of an accordion. The movement of air, going into and out of the accordion, makes a sound. This is similar to how a singer can hold a note. Pull the accordion apart, and the air moves into the device (ribs are pulled up when reaching overhead; the air moves inward upon inhale). Squeeze the accordion, and the air is pushed out (ribs move down and compress the lung space when exhaling). Some of my patients were singers, and they seemed to always know how to use the breathing muscles. You can also learn how to breathe with these movements and practice how to move air and avoid holding your breath. This strategy combines effective exhaling techniques and reminds you to breathe with your body movements while performing an activity. So, how else can you conserve energy and make your breathing work better?

Energy conservation is a practice that requires us to think through the process of an activity that we would like to accomplish, then plan on how to avoid physically "overdoing it." The first question should always be this: "How do I prevent working myself into shortness of breath and fatigue?" It seems to be in our nature to want to get a task done when we start it. When it comes to managing shortness of breath, it is not healthy to "push" ourselves and work into shortness of breath. Remember, all those muscles require oxygen to do that work. If we have a hard time getting enough oxygen to those muscles and continue to work at that pace, the oxygen level in our blood decreases. Doing so can tax the entire system. Our brains, hearts, and eyes need oxygen, too! Energy conservation helps us to develop a mindset to plan and pace ourselves. Taking the time to consider the effort that a task involves and planning ahead are the most important energy conservation strategies that you can implement. Learning to use pre-planned rest breaks, self-monitoring strategies, and breathing techniques are energy conservation strategies that can help prevent you from overdoing it; it will help you better manage shortness of breath. Most importantly, in my experience, this is a healthy strategy to guide you to improve endurance and better tolerate increasing involvement in daily activities. This is what helps to lessen that "worn out by the end of the day" feeling.

So, how do you avoid overdoing it, and when should you take a rest break? Simply put, just before you need it. It's good if you were already watching or monitoring yourself for shortness of breath or fatigue when doing something. It's great if you then acted to sit down and get your breath back before going back to the task at hand. Knowing your level of strength and when you become fatigued helps guide you for safety. I recommend that you plan ahead and then monitor the jobs or activities that you already know will cause shortness of breath or fatigue. When you pace yourself and add planned rest breaks, it is intended to rest your muscles. Your body requires less oxygen while you are resting those muscles. That means you can catch your breath quicker and move along with your activity faster. This is one of the most important concepts in minimizing shortness of breath with activity that I could share with my patients. We can use pacing with rest breaks as a guideline to improve your endurance.

From a therapist's point of view, the pacing concept is used as a safety strategy to help patients perform activities in their strength range and avoid having them work into fatigue or shortness of breath. When you work within your strength range, you are in control. When a person chooses to work into fatigue or pushes himself, he has less control. That is when bad things can happen. That is when a person can become unsteady, not think as clearly, make poor decisions, and have increased anxiety. And then what happens? We rush! This is a time when accidents or falls are more likely to occur. Performing daily activities within our strength range is a safer way to guide us and promote successful outcomes. Repeatedly working in our strength range and using planned rest breaks is also how to safely build endurance. It just requires knowing how to pace ourselves.

Pacing is when you take a task and plan how to break it up into manageable pieces that are easier to recover from. Following an effective pacing strategy can also help build your endurance. When the therapist knows you can perform a task within your strength range for a set amount of time, he can then insert a rest break. An effective pacing plan is to take a short rest break before you need it, revitalize, and then to return to the task at hand. As you would not be overdoing it, you should recover quickly. You can then quickly return to that task and repeat that same timeframe, followed by another short rest break. Repeating this task-then-rest pattern in this exact timeframe provides a safety measure to guide you toward improving endurance. It also can be used to monitor yourself for fatigue while you progress.

The therapists like to use timeframes as a way to monitor a patient's progress. This is a way to measure activity that can help guide us to safely increase a patient's performance. Let's say that one timeframe is one set of an exercise. If today you can do three sets of an exercise with rest breaks five days a week, we could reasonably expect to increase to four sets at least one time next week. Our muscles and bodies respond, making it easier, and we get stronger. Using this technique, we can progressively add more sets to the exercise or increase an activity as your tolerance improves. This is how to build your endurance. It also deals with the question of fatigue. "Why do I get so tired by the end of the day, and how can I improve upon it?"

Most of our daily activities can be measured or monitored. This can then be used as a guide to pace ourselves, minimize potential fatigue, and manage shortness of breath while doing things at home. We can measure most tasks using time, usually by seconds or minutes. Distance can be measured by how far away something is, in feet, or by a visual landmark. Output can be measured by how many things can get done; this can be done by counting (i.e. number of peeled potatoes completed). Depending on which activity is performed, you would choose one of these measurements to keep track. Once we know what causes us to become short of breath or fatigued, we can then divvy it up into smaller, more manageable bits. When we know what the manageable bits are, it can guide us on when to take a rest break. We will apply this to some everyday activities.

With all of these rest breaks, how will the job get done? Who is going to wash and peel all those potatoes by dinner time? Well, here is where we need to consider some of the virtues of a rest break. The more exhausted one becomes when performing an activity, the longer it takes to recover. The longer it takes to recover, the more we are able to talk ourselves out of doing it or completing it. If I fall behind schedule, will it cause me to worry about it? The other point is that the more one pushes oneself to overdo it, to get the job done, the more an increased demand is placed on the body, and he may be hurting himself. This is not a safe practice. If you were to try this, you would not be working within your strength range and would be more likely to leave yourself exhausted. Remember, bad things can happen when working into fatigue. The cool thing to know is that when you pace yourself, you get to take a rest break before you actually "need it." Doing so will make it where you need less time to recover. You are not taxing the system or straining yourself, and you may not need to sit down to get your breath back. You are strong and in control when going to take that rest break. When the rest breaks are short and you recover quickly, you can get right back to the task at hand, and the job will get done!

Who would ever think that you may need to take a rest break when heading toward the bathroom for a bathroom break? As an OT in homecare, I would assess my patients for bathroom accessibility needs. Did the patient need a raised toilet seat or a wall mounted grab bar in the shower? Could he safely walk to the bathroom and perform his daily needs? Some patients became short of breath while walking to the bathroom. "When you've gotta go, you gotta go!" I often heard that they were not stopping for any rest breaks. "I'll sit when I get there." For safe household mobility, I would instruct on energy conservation strategies to teach them to avoid rushing off to the bathroom. Remember, bad things can happen when you work into fatigue.

In a typical home, if the bathroom was on the first floor, an average distance from a patient's bed or chair to the toilet was about thirty feet. A pacing strategy to teach some patients would be to place an outward-facing chair halfway to the bathroom, which, for the average home, is about fifteen feet. The chair is used as a fifteen-foot marker and is there for a rest break if needed. It's to be positioned there as a marker to remind you to "STOP" there and check whether or not you're getting short of breath. Another safety consideration is that, when you go to stand up, I must verify that you are not lightheaded and that your balance is steady. If not, you would sit right back down until this cleared up. Whenever you stand from sitting or lying, stay by your seat and check your balance. Wait five seconds to check for any lightheadedness and sit if needed. This tactic should be performed every time you stand up because your blood pressure needs to "catch up" to your head during a position change. Always start this process as soon as you feel the urge to use the bathroom in order to anticipate any needed rest breaks. If the balance is good, then you proceed to walk that fifteen feet to your marker. A rest stop here, while standing, allows you to check your breathing. If you become short of breath or fatigued, you have two safe options. Sit for a short rest break on that chair you positioned for yourself, or stand still and perform your puffy cheeks breathing to get your breath back. Otherwise, you are stopping only to check whether you are getting short of breath. If not, continue and walk the next fifteen feet, or the rest of the way to the toilet.

My goal as a therapist was to help my patients get comfortable with learning how to get their breath back without sitting. It was to boost their confidence in knowing that they could be engaged in activities while standing and still maintain control of their breathing. While you are walking, the leg muscles are using up a lot of the body's oxygen at that time. So, by simply stopping those leg muscles and standing still before you get too short of breath, you could get the breath back without sitting. This is when the puffy cheeks breathing, using good technique, will move air into and out of your lungs more efficiently and help to get your breath back quicker. As in the previous example, resting at the halfway marker while on the way to the toilet allows you to feel that you have gotten your breath back. Ideally, the goal is to be in control when you get to the toilet so that you can safely sit down. You can use the puffy cheeks breathing while walking and while going to sit down.

Important points to consider: If you feel the urge to use the bathroom, don't delay. It takes extra time to pace yourself. When you go to sit down, the muscles in the legs are working hard to lower your body slowly onto the toilet. Have a full breath of air in your lungs as you begin to sit and then exhale with puffy cheeks while lowering yourself. As you begin to sit, release your breath through the puffy cheeks. This controls the exhale and lets the air out slower. Having that air in the lungs makes you feel stronger while sitting down. Not only will you sound like a flat tire, but you'll also kind of look like a tire deflating as you sit down. Puffy cheeks breathing and pacing can be used as tools to conserve your energy. However, if you have been ill and are not feeling strong or steady, be patient. If you practice caution and use these strategies, you'll get back to dashing off to the potty when your endurance improves. Until then, these are some ways to avoid having a hard landing onto the toilet because you are rushing and out of breath. These are some of the pacing strategies you can learn in order to conserve your energy while moving about the home. What if you have a doctor's appointment and are required to walk farther?

The physical therapist helps to train patients to walk safely using good balance. The patient may need to learn to use an appropriate ambulatory device, like a cane, walker, or wheelchair. In homecare, the physical therapy goal was to have the patient improve his walking distance. A typical, long-term goal was to reach two hundred to three hundred feet safely, using the proper device if needed. At that distance, it is getting to where the patient is building the stamina to get safely out of the home, see his doctors, and, hopefully, begin outpatient therapy. Physical therapists will also incorporate the energy conservation strategy of pacing to improve a patient's leg strength and endurance through exercising.

When a patient's breathing was a limiting factor for walking, I would ask the patient and physical therapists to practice how to rest before needed while standing. They would try this pacing strategy with puffy cheeks breathing and train to walk farther. In the previous example, the bathroom was thirty feet away, and that patient was stopping at fifteen feet to check or monitor his breathing status. It is the use of a predetermined distance, to check ourselves for shortness of breath or fatigue, that keeps us in control and allows us to recover quickly. If the patient is now able to walk thirty feet to the bathroom and sit on the toilet without getting short of breath, we will use thirty feet as the predetermined distance to check our breathing when going outdoors.

How can you pace yourself for distance? Try to visualize what thirty feet looks like from where you are sitting. In the previous example, the distance was thirty feet to the toilet. Otherwise, you can get a rough idea by counting your steps. For this example, sixteen steps is about equal to thirty feet (one step is about two feet long). From your chair, pick a direction that you can walk sixteen steps in, and make a mental mark of that spot. Later, do it again just to verify that distance, and remember the location of your mental marker. Practicing this helps you to gauge this by eye.

Let us say that it is thirty feet to the kitchen from your seat in one direction. Then it is about thirty feet to the back door. Gauging the distance using these landmarks will help you to monitor how far you're walking outdoors. How far down the driveway is thirty feet? Can you see it? Make a mental note and walk to that point to stop for a rest break. In a store parking lot, the width of three parking spaces is about thirty feet. After a few times of using mental markers or "landmarks" to guide the distance that you walk, it gets easier, and you start to pay attention. This is the distance you should walk and then stop to check your breathing. If beginning to get short of breath, stand still and perform your puffy cheeks breathing. While you get your breath back, check for your next landmark thirty feet away and then off you go. If you stop to check your breathing and you are not short of breath, walk to your next thirty-foot marker. As you practice this "stop, check, and rest or continue" technique, you are pacing yourself and not pushing beyond your endurance limit. This has you working safely in your strength range.

As the thirty-foot rest intervals become easier to manage, you can then increase the interval distance. If the last outing was at thirty feet, then increase by half. Go to forty-five feet. Try that for the next week or more, as needed, and then increase again by half, going to sixty feet. Following this pacing technique provides a step-by-step way to monitor and improve breathing performance while increasing your endurance (i.e. distance walked without shortness of breath or related fatigue). Well, that will work if you just want to get out and walk. But what about doing more things at home? We can learn to pace ourselves in other ways when we want to get busy doing things at home.

When back at home, what if you want to cook or do some chores? Great. Just try to avoid "overdoing- it" and pace yourself. This time we'll be using the clock to monitor how long you work before taking a rest. Let's use washing dishes as an example. Your family of four finishes up dinner, and you have offered to wash the dishes. "Oh no, my dear," they say. "You've been ill, so we can wash the dishes." Sound familiar? When you are feeling better and wish to engage in activities that you had been previously active with before, it is time to start setting goals to resume those chores. Initially, set up the tasks for yourself using a family member's or helper's assistance as needed. That would be planning ahead and using an important energy conservation strategy. It would be wise to communicate your intentions with your family in preparation. Working together with them initially can help you succeed and may also reassure them of your abilities. Ask that your helper move the dishes to the sink, and you can wash them. Good goal. Nice strategy! Now, how to pace yourself and be safe?

Let's use time as your next pacing strategy to monitor yourself while washing the dishes. You can use the clock. In the kitchen and near the sink, turn a chair out so that you will have a spot to rest when needed. When ready, note the time and go to the sink. Wash dishes for two minutes and then stop. Check your breathing and fatigue level. If starting to get short of breath or fatigued, then start puffy cheeks breathing and go to sit in your chair. After a short break that allows you to recover quickly, check the clock and return to the sink for two more minutes of washing dishes. Repeat the two-minute intervals and then rest. As you engage in tasks while using time as the pacing strategy, you are monitoring for fatigue before you need a rest break. When you feel as though you can go longer, add another minute to your dishwashing time before resting. Increase the time in one-minute increments as your endurance improves.

Another pacing strategy uses output or "number of tasks" completed. Monitor your fatigue level by using the number of items completed before taking a rest. Let's go back to the kitchen and plan this out. As previously mentioned, know where you will sit to rest and prepare this area near your workstation (i.e. turn a chair out at the table and assure a clear walkway in the kitchen). This time we are going to help prepare the meal. What is the goal? Wash, peel, and cut some potatoes. We're having a roast tonight! You will certainly want to discuss your meal preparation plan with your helpers. Also, communicate with them any set-up needs. Perhaps the potatoes are in a hopper down in the basement. Ask to have those potatoes brought up to the kitchen counter. This will save steps, literally, while you are looking quite savvy in your planning. Planning ahead is the number one energy conservation technique. Planning out your job and discussing it with your helpers avoids unnecessary steps. After you have set up your food-prep area for peeling potatoes, decide how many it takes to feed your family of four. You know they love your potatoes. So, let's prepare eight medium-sized potatoes.

Using the pacing strategy of number of tasks, start off easy and attempt to complete a two-item task. Initially, remember to start with fewer tasks so that you can recover quickly with a rest break. Let's break up those tasks. Stand up and move to the kitchen sink. Pull eight potatoes from the bag, inspect them, and place them next to the sink = one task (put any bad potatoes in the sink; it's a separate task to throw them out). Ensure that you have a scrubbing pad and utensils for cleaning and cutting = one task. Stop and stand still. Check for shortness of breath or fatigue. If short of breath, begin puffy cheeks breathing. You will soon be attempting to get your breath back by simply standing still while using this breathing technique. If fatigued, however, return to your seat for a short rest break. When rested, return to the kitchen counter and scrub two potatoes = two tasks. Again, you will then check your breathing and determine if a rest is needed due to fatigue. Repeat this pacing strategy until all the potatoes are peeled. By using the "number of tasks" strategy as a guide, you can monitor yourself and know when to use a rest break. As your endurance improves, strengthen yourself by adding an additional task and work at that level until you are ready to advance. You may be able to advance by one or two tasks each week. This is another way to gauge your performance in steps in order to help safely guide yourself in progressing your endurance level.

Pacing yourself helps to prevent shortness of breath and working into fatigue, and it provides a guide to improving your endurance. The strategic use of rest breaks is paramount to conserving your energy and progressing. A rest break infers that there is a job to get done or a task to complete. Please do not view taking rest breaks as "being lazy." Stopping at intervals lets you check yourself for shortness of breath or fatigue while under control (in your strength range). The timely use of rest breaks lets you recover quickly so that you can get back to the task at hand. The goal is to progress and build your endurance while not beating yourself up when trying to get there. The practice of applying these strategies with successful outcomes is what will help you to build confidence in your abilities.

While setting yourself up to be successful, be careful, especially early on in your recovery. Plan to use helpers for assistance. Assure proper use of prescribed medications and oxygen. Pay attention to your diet. Plan ahead. For example, if using oxygen, know how many cylinders should be taken to the doctor's office and know how to carry them. Many facilities have wheelchairs that can tote cylinders. Call in advance for availability. Err to the side of safety. As you get stronger, you will achieve your goal of greater independence and improve your confidence in managing shortness of breath.

IV

Improve Your Confidence, Know Your Limits

Breathing exercises improve the correct muscular parts of breathing. Puffy cheeks breathing improves exhaling efficiency by moving more of the bad air out so that when you breathe back in, the fresh air has somewhere to go. Learning to take advantage of breathing with your body movements helps you move air in and out of the lungs. Conserving your energy has you planning ahead so you don't waste your breath. Every therapist will tell you that the more you practice, the easier it gets. That is how to progress. Using the training that the therapists provide you as a guide can help you build confidence in your abilities. Generally, as soon as people see that something works for them and it helps, they are going to do that again. As you practice these breathing instructions, it will help to build your confidence. Know that if or when you become short of breath while engaged in an activity, you have learned some strategies that will help you get it back.

When our health is with us, we are all confident in our breathing. It is when dealing with a heart, lung, or other medical condition that our confidence in relying on our breathing may be shaken. If we can regain that confidence, it puts us in a more relaxed state while we manage our daily activities. This breathe to function program is designed to help improve your understanding of the components that lead to shortness of breath with activity, along with how to treat it. My goal is to show you that, with improved confidence in your ability to manage shortness of breath, you will be better able to relax should a stressful event occur. Nothing can be more anxiety-provoking than getting short of breath and having difficulty getting it back.

Anxiety places the entire body in a heightened state of tension. If unable to relax, we may feel at a loss of control. That tension may also trigger or perpetuate pain responses. In response to heightened muscular tension, we can develop patterns of ineffective shallow or rapid breathing. Along with making it difficult to relax, tension also increases the demand for oxygen in the body. I pointed out earlier how more oxygen is used by the leg muscles if we keep walking than if we just stand still to relax. If unable to relax due to anxiety, that tension can also use up more oxygen than a breathing-compromised person may be able to provide. This is often when we hear that a person could not get their breath back, and they either had to be taken to the hospital or summon the emergency medical system (EMS).

A key thing to remember is that if you know you can do something to reduce anxiety and relax during a stressful event, you can minimize the stress on the breathing system and better manage a stress-inducing occurrence. As your OT, I want you to learn how to cope and prepare yourself to recover from the activities or events that may bring about shortness of breath. If there is one thing you should remember when shortness of breath develops, it's to STOP what you are doing and breathe! To help relax yourself, use the puffy cheeks breathing technique you have been practicing. It's a shallow breather preventer! Try to remember to use this technique if stressed or anxious, and do it as fast as your breathing at that time. This technique aims to improve the efficiency of moving the bad air out and bringing fresh air back into your lungs. As this is practiced and implemented, it can help you to gain confidence in knowing that you can help yourself. If you can remain calm and relaxed during a stressful event, it can help you to maintain that control and, hopefully, return to your relaxed state. Please keep your physician up to date with any new anxiety-related symptoms and notify him if any breathing difficulties persist or worsen.

Now that you are learning these breathing techniques and how to exercise the muscles for breathing, let's learn how to apply it to more challenging daily activities. As previously instructed, before you start an activity, think to yourself, "When do I stop to check my breathing?" This planning-ahead strategy helps you to know your limits and keeps you from doing too much so that you can recover more quickly. Again, as our bodies move, they are using more oxygen. Our lungs, however, may not be sufficiently moving oxygen into the bloodstream to meet the demands of our bodies. The brain will sense the oxygen-to-blood-transfer needs and increase the respiratory rate to get more air in and out of the lungs. If we are engaged in an activity and we know that point where the breathing starts to get faster, we can identify that as the redline. A redline is a point at which an activity should stop; it helps us to know our limits. If we know that redline, we can avoid overly stressing our bodies. We can then take a quick break from the activity and use that break to check our status. This is a key moment to be aware of when using my instruction. This helps you to avoid working into fatigue while maintaining control. Knowing your redline and how to respond is another energy conservation strategy. It is a plan that looks to help you conserve your energy by minimizing fatigue so that you can better make it through the day.

The alternative to knowing your redline and when to "stop, check, and rest" is continuing to keep going until you are exhausted. I have had patients who would become very anxious with their breathing. Without knowing about other strategies to help them, they would try to do what they could when they could. These were the folks who would press ahead and just keep going until they got to where they were going, or until the job was done. This strategy can deprive the body of oxygen, and they worked to exhaustion. At that point, it becomes much harder on us and takes longer to recover from that job or activity. This is working past the redline, which continuously stresses the body. Performing activities in this fashion will leave us in a constant state of fatigue. This is not the way to do things and expect to make it through the day.

To the best of your ability, resist the urge to rush back and try to engage in the activities that used to be easily accomplished. Bring your activity level up as you feel comfortable. Pacing yourself and using the breathing techniques are the tools to apply for your next job.

The so-called jobs that comprise our days are basically…everything! Whether it's walking around the house, baking a potato casserole, or taking out the trash. Our goal should be this: "I want to do what I would like to get done and not beat myself up trying to get there." We should try to avoid that worn-out-by-the-end-of-the-day feeling. I tell my patients that repetition of these instructed pacing strategies within their strength range or comfortable range is the technique that can improve that feeling.

We have already learned of ways to breathe with our body movements while reaching, bending, and walking. Now let's learn to breathe with exertion. The first rule of managing shortness of breath is this: Do not hold your breath! Therapists are always watching patients breathing patterns' as they perform their exercises. It is especially important. When we exert ourselves, like when lifting a heavy weight, we are often inclined to breathe in to the fullest extent and hold it as we lift. Perhaps we feel it prepares us for the load and makes us feel stronger. It does seem easier when we contract our muscles around an air-filled rib cage. Doing this does provide rigidity and stability in the upper trunk while we perform some feat of strength, exercise, or heavy activity. It makes us feel stronger. The problem with this is that if we continue to hold our breath, we are straining ourselves at that time.

Holding your breath while exerting can build up pressure within your body. Using this tactic may lead to a variety of internal injuries. You're likely to just "pop." A safer technique is to always test the load and to breathe with the exertion.

There is something to be said about performing a feat of strength with our lungs and rib cage filled with air. It does make us feel stronger. The safe way to do this, though, is by knowing when to breathe and not holding your breath while exerting. The pattern or "formula" for safe breathing while exerting ourselves is this: Take a nice full breath of air in through the nose, or both nose and mouth, and perform the exertion task while blowing out the mouth with puffy cheeks. Keep the exertion time short.

Let's use weightlifting as an example. Let's say you were able to lift twenty-five pounds over your head and hold it there. After testing the load to ensure you can still pick up twenty-five pounds, breathe in fully and exert to push the weight up while exhaling with puffy cheeks. With the weight overhead, the exertion part will occur while you lower the weight. Breathe in fully and exhale using puffy cheeks while lowering the weight. Now, that's breathing properly with exertion. So, how do we breathe with the activities that exert us at home? Try using that formula!

Let's look at a routine task that requires you to exert yourself, like moving from sitting in an armchair to standing. When moving from sitting to standing, you exert yourself the moment you push off from the chair. The point at which you exert the most of your energy is when you use your legs to lift your butt off the seat and come to standing. Let us learn to apply the exertion formula and breathe with this task. Use puffy cheeks breathing while you reposition your hips at the front edge of the seat. This is the spot on the chair that you should stand up from and sit back down onto. As you lean forward to shift your weight and position your head out over the knees, breathe in fully and comfortably. As the lungs become filled and your head is out over the knees, push down on the armrests and exert with your legs to come to standing, blowing out with puffy cheeks as you come to standing. This takes advantage of the strength we feel throughout the rib cage and upper body when the lungs are filled with air. Not only do we feel stronger doing it, but we are also safely adding the breathing to the task. To sit back down, reverse the procedure. Breathe in. When the lungs feel near full capacity, bend at the hips and knees and bring your head out over your knees. Reach for the armrests and lower yourself while blowing out with puffy cheeks. Now, that is breathing with your body movements. Can we breathe like that while climbing stairs?

More than likely, climbing up the stairs is the number one activity in the home that, when we exert ourselves, will cause shortness of breath. If the assessment was needed, the physical therapists would determine when our patients in homecare were safe to stair climb. They would monitor breathing and fatigue levels while teaching the patient and caregivers how to climb steps, all while considering any surgical precautions or ambulatory devices, and then provide any necessary equipment recommendations. When the patient was safe to stair climb using the provided physical therapy instruction, the occupational therapist would reinforce that stair climbing instruction while going to assess for any needs in the upstairs bathroom, upstairs bedroom, or downstairs laundry room.

The occupational therapist would then assess the patient's bathroom for accessibility, durable medical equipment (DME) needs, and safe set-up for the performance of hygiene needs while upstairs. The OT also assesses the bedroom for safety regarding bed positioning, transfers, dressing, and any clothing retrieval needs. The basement would also be assessed, when ready, for safety in performing laundry or obtaining supplies from the pantry. A patient's strength and endurance are important performance components that are assessed during activities in those parts of the home. While performing a variety of routine activities, we could see if a patient's breathing and fatigue levels would impact his performance during those tasks. Early on in his recovery process, tasks that exerted the patient needed to be considered during their day. Those activities add up. To conserve energy, we'd instruct on how to know his limits and be safe. The training would help to answer questions regarding how to be prepared: Am I strong enough for this task, or do I need a helper? Is there a chair at the top of the steps? Where will I sit to rest? Will my oxygen line reach all the way upstairs? Is there a walker at the top of the stairs? For now, let us focus on the completion of one task upstairs. Incorporate what you've learned about pacing, monitoring breathing and fatigue and using those rest breaks. Let's go upstairs.

Patients and caregivers are often instructed by the therapists on how the breathing is impacted while stair climbing. When we look at stair climbing, one of the more difficult parts of the task, for our patient, is the exertion required for one leg (the good leg) to lift the body up to the next step. You can utilize the exertion formula for breathing while stair climbing. Begin by puffy cheeks breathing as you walk to the stairs and reach for the hand-rail. With your hand on the railing, place your foot on the first step (use the good leg). That's not too difficult. The hard part is getting the other foot up onto that step. Using the exertion formula, start breathing in when you move the first foot onto the step, and as the lungs become filled with air, push down with that same leg and pull on the rail as you bring the other foot up, all while exhaling with puffy cheeks. Check your breathing. If you are becoming short of breath, stand still and puffy cheeks breathe until you get your breath back. If you are too short of breath with one step, reconsider stair climbing at this time, at least until your endurance improves. If they are unaware of this, let your doctors know about how this breathing difficulty occurs. The physical therapist may need to guide you further with the stair climbing safety instruction.

If the breathing is manageable, you will repeat the previous breathe-with-exertion procedure for climbing the next step. To conserve your energy and plan ahead, choose to use every fourth step as your rest stop. Stand there to monitor yourself, and if needed, get your breath back before proceeding. If you are fatigued and must rest, you can turn to sit on the steps. While holding one handrail with both hands, turn around and sit on the second step up from the step you are on. That will be the step closer to your butt as you sit Use your puffy cheeks breathing to exhale as you sit. Your helper can guide you. Together, you can decide if you have the endurance to continue going upstairs, as it may require too much exertion at this time.

Another activity that frequently requires us to exert ourselves is when having a bowel movement. There may be times when you have constipation or difficulty emptying the bowels. Some folks would sit down, hold their breath, and push hard. This has us straining ourselves and builds up internal pressure, which is not a safe practice. Building up internal pressure while straining is also a safety concern for women during childbirth. They are taught a technique called Lamaze breathing. This technique has them breathing with the exertion of pushing during the birthing process. Similarly, a safe way to avoid straining while relieving oneself would be to breathe with the diaphragm while using some forethought.

Now, let's learn to avoid a straining injury while exerting to have a bowel movement. If you've sat on the toilet and nothing is moving, don't fight it! Get up and leave the bathroom. Try using proven strategies that you know work or that were recommended to you by your doctor in order to avoid and manage constipation. Ensure you are taking in adequate fluids. Prune juice can be used to help with regularity. Eating foods with fiber has also been known to improve regularity. Laxatives provide varying levels of relief. If constipation has not been addressed in the past, ask your doctor for guidance. Ensure that your doctor is aware of your current laxative preparations and verify that they are safe to take with any newer medications you may have been prescribed recently.

When a person is confronted with a new or ongoing medical condition, other factors can affect the regularity of the bowels. Appetite or diet changes that may occur while recuperating and not feeling well can affect normal regularity. Those appetite changes may lead to not drinking adequately or making unhealthy food choices. We also must consider that a patient's activity level has been diminished and that he can become more sedentary during his recovery. He may not be getting the muscular activity that promotes a healthy gut, such as bending, twisting, reaching, and walking, during his illness. A good therapist would tell you that daily diet and exercise promote healthy bowel patterns. Well, that therapist would be right. Until then, there are several methods to utilize to minimize constipation. As the diet considerations, preparations, and mother nature take their course, you will find yourself back in the bathroom and ready to go. Here you can apply the breathing with exertion formula and coordinate safe breathing with a bowel movement.

If you are not doing this already, try to learn how to use your diaphragm muscle with breathing; it can help prevent overexerting during a bowel movement. The shape of the diaphragm muscle is like a flat plate that rests above the stomach. When you inhale, it moves downward and pushes your tummy outward. Let us use what we've learned with exercise #3: The diaphragm breathing exercise, along with breathing fully, will help empty the bowels.

After you have prepared yourself and you are sitting on the toilet, fold your arms across your belly, lean forward, and rest your arms on your thighs. This position with help you go. If you have too much belly, cup your hands under the tummy where it meets the top of your legs, then lean forward. When you lean forward, your arms or hands will push back into your tummy, as they are blocked by your thighs. While in this position, you are blocking your tummy with your arms in a comfortable position. When ready, breathe in fully. Because you now are experienced at diaphragm breathing (ex. #3) and are a better belly breather, you will feel your tummy pushing into your arms as you inhale fully. The position of your arms or hands will block that outward movement of the tummy and give those abdominal muscles something to push against. During a full inhale, the tummy's movement outward is blocked by your arms, and they resist the tummy from pushing outward. The diaphragm movement will then assist in pushing downward, in the direction you are trying to relieve yourself. Breathe in fully to expand the lungs with your tummy; this will push the diaphragm downward. When the lungs are nearly full, push to exert your bowels, then relax and exhale with puffy cheeks. The tummy pushing outward against your folded arms provides some "gut leverage" and assists with the pushing process. In the end, this has you breathing to help push while going to the bathroom. It helps you to avoid holding your breath while exerting and prevents too much pressure from building up within your body.

These are examples of how we may exert ourselves with daily activities. The breathing with exertion formula shows how to breathe in fully, exert yourself, and then quickly relax with an exhale so that you can work within your abilities and avoid a straining type of injury. This technique can be applied to all activities that you may find yourself straining to complete. These are energy conservation strategies I would teach as a part of an occupational therapy care plan so that you could safely complete daily activities, conserve your energy, and make it through the day.

What if all that daytime activity does not earn you a good night's sleep? Oftentimes, the anxieties formed from dealing with shortness of breath or other daily stressors do not turn off when it comes to the end of the day and it's time to sleep. I have shown you that this breathing program helps us to get through the day; can it help us rest through the night? Why yes, it can!

Relaxation breathing. I think the Chinese get credit for discovering its benefits a thousand years ago. We keep recycling those benefits of breathing for relaxation and calling them our own. The reality is, if we can improve upon our breathing using strategies that do a better job of getting oxygen into the blood, it has a calming effect. So why not try using puffy cheeks breathing for relaxation? When puffy cheeks breathing is practiced here, it often gets us to yawn or heavy sigh. I would frequently observe this while instructing my patients, and have felt this myself. That is when I know it's working right. See if you notice this happening to you while practicing. It also helps you to find a comfortable, relaxed state of breathing. Let's use it now to help fall asleep.

Safety consideration: Please be aware of the importance of using prescribed oxygen or ventilation-assisted devices such as a CPAP or BiPAP at night. These must be used at night, as they were prescribed by the doctor for a reason. When irregular breathing occurs at night, it is unmonitored. While sleeping, way too much time can get by if not breathing properly. This is a time when oxygen depletion can occur and lower the blood oxygen levels. You may not sense this, and it can occur without warning. The long-term effects of this can be seriously detrimental. The CPAP and BiPAP provide ventilation assistance through a mask. Once you become used to wearing the mask and your oxygen needs are met, this alone can relax your body for a good night's sleep. If you have one and are not used to it or are unable to relax, notify the equipment provider. They will have a mask that can fit your needs. Trial and error fittings are often required. Puffy cheeks breathing may not work here due to the positioning of the different types of face masks. An oxygen concentrator is a machine that delivers the oxygen through a nasal cannula (nose tubes) or a face mask. Puffy cheeks breathing can be practiced with these devices.

When it is time to fall asleep, it never fails that, once we lie down, we start thinking about the whole world. That brain activity, along with those thoughts that get stirred up, does not help us to doze off. If you are lying there thinking about everything, it's quite possible you are shallow breathing at that time. That is when a relaxation strategy helps to shift your focus back onto your sleeping and, hopefully, take your mind off other matters. I believe that is why people used to count sheep. That was an old sleep strategy that refocused one's attention back on himself by counting—a diversion technique that attempted to shift oneself from stress-inducing thoughts.

As you practice your puffy cheeks breathing and the technique improves, you will gain confidence in using it as a tool to help your breathing and using it to relax. Try using this as a sleep strategy. As you lie in bed comfortably, your breath rate normally slows down. This is because your body is not moving; the muscles require less oxygen. If you lie down and are not falling asleep in five minutes or so, try using the puffy cheeks breathing as a relaxation tool. This helps to slow the breath rate while moving air in and out of the lungs. Because you are not physically moving very much, it feels comfortable to breathe low and slow; your body is not asking to breathe fast. At that time, it may feel comfortable to go longer with your breaths and take up to three seconds to breathe in and six seconds to breathe out. You will find that, with the slower, relaxed breaths and the better transfer of air that puffy cheeks breathing provides, shallow breathing will be minimized, and it can help you to relax. You may start to yawn or sigh and relax enough to better fall asleep. I would encourage my patients to practice this natural relaxation strategy to help them with sleeping. This breathing technique simply helps to get more oxygen into the bloodstream, and when it gets to the brain, it has a calming effect. Personally, if I cannot fall asleep after five minutes and I wish to, I always use the puffy cheeks breathing. It helps me to relax and take my mind off other matters, putting the focus on falling asleep (See YouTube video [PCB] relaxing to fall asleep). The other technique I use to help me fall asleep is to refocus and think of music as a diversion. Use one of your favorite soft songs or ballads. I use the song "Dust in the Wind" by Kansas. Singing softly or saying your prayers also helps to move air into and out of your lungs if shallow breathing is keeping you awake. Be sure to notify your doctor if sleeping is difficult, as there may be other issues affecting your sleep patterns.

The environment within our homes must also be considered as potentially having an impact on our breathing. How long have the windows been closed for the hot or cold weather seasons? What type of allergens are prevalent either inside or outside of the home? Who knows where all the dust comes from? Is your area clean? It makes sense to keep track of airborne irritants like perfumes, air fresheners, candles, and fumes from household cleaners. Ensure timely replacement of furnace filters and routine maintenance of heating, ventilation, and air conditioning (HVAC) systems.

Heat and humidity can also impact your breathing and fatigue levels. It pays to watch the weatherman and plan accordingly. When going out to see the doctor, get the car ready to better accommodate your breathing needs. For example, park in the shade, or use the air conditioner to cool the car, which removes humidity.

As a homecare therapist, it seemed that one of the activities that often led to shortness of breath and fatigue was bathing. It makes sense. You are working in a confined area of high humidity and heat. Even though the heated water feels good, that heat combined with the humidity from the shower can influence both breathing and fatigue levels. To manage this, start off with the basics. If you have a bathroom ventilation fan, turn it on as soon as you turn on the shower or tub faucet. If you are without a fan and it is warm outside, partially open the window. Otherwise, leave the bathroom door a quarter of the way open to allow the steam and humidity to escape. If you use oxygen, be sure to use it while bathing or showering. You will be doing plenty of reaching and scrubbing while you bathe. This activity has your body requiring an increased amount of oxygen.

While bathing, steam and humidity put moisture into the air. This moisture competes with the oxygen going into your lungs. The other part is to plan ahead to conserve your energy during the task. If you stand to shower, you may want to consider a tub seat or shower chair. Sitting to shower is quite relaxing and allows your leg muscles to rest. I believe sitting to shower has a huge energy conservation benefit, especially if balance safety is a concern. A handheld shower allows you to redirect the spray so that you are not getting hit in the face with the water. A hand-shower works particularly well when using a tub seat. If you do not have a hand-shower, adjust the shower head to one side (the wall side).

Try to avoid bathing or showering when you are tired. If your peak energy level is after breakfast, shower then. Avoid waiting until evening, as you may be more fatigued. Remember, bad things happen when you work while fatigued. It is also safe practice to shower when someone is in the home. Otherwise, take a phone into the bathroom and place it near the tub or shower, within reach, so you'll have it if an emergency arises. Use the instruction from chapter three: Breathe with your body movements when reaching above and below your waist while bathing. Check your breathing at intervals and use puffy cheeks breathing with short rest breaks to prevent working yourself into fatigue or shortness of breath. Structure your day to have time to rest after bathing. This is planning ahead to conserve your energy. What about doing more difficult tasks, like household chores?

Following a hospitalization or a major medical procedure, patients are often placed on light-duty status at the onset of their recovery process. That means participating in light, day-to-day activities as tolerated, such as eating, dressing, light-meal preparation, and walking short distances. Those activities may require some occupational therapy for instruction. Sometimes bathing and stair climbing will require assistance or further instruction. Other household chores, such as vacuuming, sweeping and mopping, laundry, window cleaning, and putting fitted sheets on the bed, are considered heavy homemaking tasks. Give yourself time to get stronger and develop your breathing skills prior to engaging in the heavy homemaking tasks or chores. Oftentimes, it requires the doctor's prior approval to resume heavy homemaking activities. If possible, recruit the assistance of family and friends, or hire a helper to assist you with completing the scheduled, heavy homemaking jobs. As your breathing and fatigue become better managed and you feel stronger, start back slowly. At first, try to do one of the easier heavy homemaking tasks, like sweeping or doing a light load of laundry if the washing machine is easily accessible.

For sweeping, as discussed in chapter three, use the pacing strategy: use distance to conserve your energy and break the task up into more manageable pieces. For a moderately sized kitchen of fifteen-by-fifteen feet, sweep one quarter of the kitchen floor. Then stop, check your breathing, and sit to rest if needed. Remember, you are trying to stay ahead of fatigue so that the rest breaks are shorter and you're not overdoing it. Complete the sweeping with rest breaks, going by one-quarter intervals. Break this task up further with a larger kitchen or one with lots of nooks and crannies.

If the laundry is on the first floor, a light load of laundry can be performed. Be sure to use your breathing techniques when bending and reaching while using the washer and dryer (see chapter three: reaching into kitchen cabinets). It may be easier to fold the few items you have while standing at a countertop or table. Try to keep supplies within reach, such as laundry soap and a basket. Choose a pacing technique to monitor your breath rate and fatigue level, such as counting number of tasks (ex: fold two towels and then check your breathing for shortness of breath; rest if needed).

As your endurance improves after a week or two, add another heavy homemaking chore to the list. Save vacuuming for last, as this takes a lot of energy. It's nice to recruit helpers for some of the heavier jobs at home. This will free you up to do more of the things you would rather be doing. As your appetite improves, how about making a full meal or baking your therapists some cookies.

An important point to consider, as discussed earlier, is adequate nutrition and hydration. We all must eat and drink to regain and maintain good health. For some, it requires following a doctor recommended diet. Ugh! That's okay. There are ways to be creative with food preparation, even when following doctor guidelines. If you are not feeling creative or you don't claim to be a cooking channel expert, find the cooks or "foodies" of the family and ask for suggestions. Creative ideas can be found for any meal plan or diet regimen. Sometimes it does take more than one cook in the kitchen to make some good down-home cooking. Also, cooking is a wonderful activity that is engaging and can be utilized to help build your endurance. Use your energy conservation strategies to perform the tasks. Monitor your breathing and pace yourself.

When we eat, it is important to consider that the amount of food in the stomach can cause us to feel short of breath. That bloated feeling we sometimes get after eating a full meal is due to the stomach filling up. The stomach is positioned below the diaphragm. If the stomach is full, the diaphragm movement can be restricted. This may, in fact, make breathing more difficult. In chapter two, we talked about how important it is to use the diaphragm. It is the number one muscle for breathing. One effective strategy for managing any breathing restriction from a bloated stomach is eating smaller portions more often during the day.

I would often have experiences with patients who went the other way. They came home from the hospitals with little or no appetite! We had to come up with strategies to get them to eat. The doctors would tell them to eat smaller portions throughout the day, and we called these portions "mini-meals." Well, if we normally eat three meals per day, eating half that meal and spreading it throughout the day will get you six mini-meals per day. This is a simple way to limit the amount of food in the stomach at any one time. It can also be used to encourage a picky eater. That sounds easy enough. Sure, and then you'll hear, "I'm not going to eat six times a day! I don't eat that much!"

In homecare, most folks came home with dietary or nutritional instructions from the doctor. If you have not received any dietary instruction, ask your doctor if diet intake instruction is needed. We would worry that our patients might not eat or drink enough. It is imperative to know which type of foods you should eat and how much food and water you should consume daily. That information provides a guideline and allows you to monitor your daily intake. Having to contend with shortness of breath is stressful on the body. Our bodies use up more energy to compensate for this increased effort. A change in appetite can have a serious effect on meeting our daily nutritional or fluid needs. Because of this, we sometimes see patients readmitted into the hospital due to malnutrition or dehydration. This can occur quickly and requires close monitoring. Let's talk about eating strategies for when you're home following an illness or if you have appetite changes.

If your appetite has been poor or eating has left you feeling overly full, try a different type of pacing strategy. If you can sit down to a nutritionally-balanced meal, try eating half of it and save the other half to eat later. It does, however, take some effort to stay on track using this mini-meal dinner strategy. Using the half-meals strategy will alter eating times during the day. If your first of six mini-meals starts at 9:00 a.m., then to stay on schedule, it will be time to nibble on something again by 11:00 a.m. The nurses call this "grazing," a term they use for when you eat small portions throughout the day. This type of eating schedule would have you eating a mini-meal at 9:00 a.m., 11:00 a.m., 1:00 p.m., 3:00 p.m., 5:00 p.m., and 7:00 p.m. Eating something or grazing every other hour throughout the day will keep you on pace to meet your nutritional needs. As you are eating less at each mealtime, it is especially important to keep up with the six mini-meal schedule. Use notes as reminders, or ask your helper to keep track of this type of eating schedule.

If not doing so already, keep track of nutritional amounts by reading the nutrition facts label that is placed on every food package. The most helpful facts are shown at the top of the label. The two that are most important to consider here are: how much one serving size equals (i.e. one half cup dry, 40 grams); and number of calories per serving (i.e. oatmeal has 150 calories per serving) (FDA).

The USDA government dietary guidelines help to keep us on track in meeting our daily nutritional needs. The USDA recommends a daily calorie intake of 1,800 calories for women and 2,400 calories for men (USDA). These are for all moderately active people of average size and everyone over fifty-one years of age (For men, this is reduced to 2,200 calories at age sixty-six). For a woman, that comes to about 300 calories per mini-meal, and it's 400 calories for men. See Table 1 to calculate calories per serving size for breakfast. When determining which food has how many calories, look at the serving size first. These are nutritional values you will find written on every package. You can visit your own pantry and read the nutritional labels located on the foods that you like.

Table 1 - Breakfast items

Serving size	Item	Calories
½ cup	Plain oatmeal	150
4 ounces	Yogurt	75
1 cup	Milk - 2%	129
1	Egg	72
1 cup	Orange juice	115
1	Banana	134
2 ounces	Ham	128
1 patty	Sausage	92
2 Tablespoons	Peanut butter	188
1.5 ounces	Cheese	60

When helping my patient learn about safe diet intake and meal scheduling strategies, I would always make reference to "the serving sizes" because, when it comes to the USDA government guidelines, a so-called "healthy plate" does not have a lot on it (USDA-how much, MyPlate).

This has always been a helpful edge in getting someone with a poor appetite to eat. I recommend portioning out a serving size when presenting food or drink to any picky eater. That would be anyone with a decreased appetite or anyone who is following a mini-meals schedule. When portioned out and positioned on a plate, the quantity of a single serving size does not look like that much (i.e. four ounces of yogurt, two ounces of ham, one cup of grapes, two Tbsp of peanut butter). If possible, provide portioned amounts to avoid that visually overwhelmed response: "I can't eat all of that!" This strategy may also encourage the poor drinker. An eight-ounce cup of water is less overwhelming to look at than a thirty-two-ounce jug when placed in front of him. It is recommended that we drink six to eight, eight-ounce servings of fluid per day. I would encourage my patients to drink at least half of this as water, if possible. Use this every-other-hour strategy if scheduled drinking helps to keep you on track. Alternating the drinking and eating schedules may also help (i.e. 9:00 a.m. eat, 10:00 a.m. drink, and so on). Portioning the sizes may also make it easier to keep track. Bigger is not always better; smaller and more often may be more helpful in meeting your nutritional intake goals.

Some of the foods we eat are better at "sticking" with us while offering "good calories." Mostly, this includes foods with protein. Foods like meat, cheese, eggs, milk, seafood, beans, yogurt, peanut butter, and oatmeal are all higher in protein. (See Table 2) The Food and Nutrition Board, Institute of Medicine, National Academies (2012) recommends the daily protein intake for adults, which is fifty-six grams for male and forty-six grams for female.

It helped to encourage my picky eaters, as, for the most part, these foods are often well liked. What is important is the fact that our bodies require that protein for daily cell growth and healing. Protein also helps the blood carry oxygen throughout the body (Piedmont Healthcare). If you or your loved one has little appetite, it is helpful to try and steer you or this person toward the foods that are higher in protein. A simple snack that I always encouraged was peanut butter on toast. The kids love this one, and if you haven't tried it, it's tasty and easy. The other thing I encouraged was to hard-boil half a dozen eggs; it's convenient, and they can be kept in the refrigerator for a quick protein punch.

Many people will try to eat "healthy" by eating mostly fruit, vegetables, and bread. Many of those foods are lacking in protein and may just feel more filling. They do provide good sources of fiber, which is helpful for the bowels. When these foods are well liked, just try to add a little protein to go with them (pre-cut cheese, cottage cheese, yogurt, or a serving of milk). Here are some vegetables and bread with higher protein amounts (See Table 3).

In trying to keep meals simple and affordable, all the foods listed in these tables are considered staples and can usually be found in most home pantries. Staples are generally the foods we like and already have on hand. These are what we purchase regularly at the grocery store. A part of meal prep is planning ahead. It is a good way to take a task that you may already know and utilize it to help get yourself back to being involved with an everyday, "normal" activity.

Table 2

Amount (serving size)	High protein sources — Item	Protein (grams)
2 ounces	Tuna canned- water	10
2 ounces	Tuna canned- oil	14
3 ounces	Yellowfin tuna	25
3 ounces	Chicken- skinless	28
3 ounces	Steak	26
3 ounces	Pork	22
3 ounces	Turkey- roasted	25
¼ cup	Lentils	11
2 Tbsp	Peanut butter	7
1 large	Egg	6
1 slice (21 grams)	Cheese	3
1 cup, (8 oz.)	2% Milk	8
6 ounces	2% Yogurt-plain (Greek)	17
½ cup (dry)	Oatmeal	5

Table 3

Amount	Vegetable/bread Protein sources	Protein (grams)
1 ear	Corn	4.7
1	Artichoke	5.3
1	Potato	3.1
1 cup	Avocado	2.9
2 Tbsp	Hummus	2.0
1 slice	Bread	2.0

Use the grocery store circulars and advertisements to help plan ahead for what you like and what supplies you may be low on. Construct a grocery store list using any dietary guidelines from your doctor, USDA guidelines for daily nutritional recommendations, and good sales. To me, there is nothing better than planning your own meals and cooking something tasty in the kitchen. Playing this numbers game certainly gets you thinking. If that doesn't light you up, recruit a family member to help you add up your numbers and meal plan. It not only has you focusing on your health through nutritional intake, but it also may bring more awareness to your family members' diet patterns, as well. They may appreciate your looking after their wellbeing. Getting yourself back into that kind of meal planning may stir some memories of old family recipes. If your family is supportive of it, that may encourage you to get back to cooking, as well. The heart of most homes is in the kitchen.

We may be inclined to use meal supplements like Ensure or Boost. These items are used to supplement the meals if an appetite is poor, but they are expensive. I tell most folks to just go to their pantry! Most of us already have the staples on hand that can meet our nutritional needs. If you are in need or are just considering the use of a supplement, ask your doctor which would be recommended. They will advise you on any meal supplement needs and provide you with safe guidelines for their use. There are many types to consider, patients have different needs, and there are many to choose from. I wish you good health and a good appetite. Good luck.

In completing this book, I realize there is a lot of information presented. I will include a condensed version or a "cheat sheet" for the person who does not wish to read all the intricacies of how an OT would treat shortness of breath. Please use the cheat sheet as a guide and reference to the book as needed. The cheat sheet will have the exercise handout, along with important safety and energy conservation strategies to consider during activities. Page numbers will be provided to help you to find those subjects inside the book. If you have further medical questions, I will ask you to inquire with your doctor. For questions related to my book, I can be reached via email at ckmiecikot@gmail.com.

Thank you.

Chris Kmiecik, OTR/L

V

Conclusion

My goal for writing this book was twofold. I wanted to share the strategies that I applied in my patient care as an occupational therapist with everybody who may be dealing with breathing issues. These breathing strategies came about through my training as a therapist, through experiences while working with some fine pulmonary and rehabilitation specialists, and while working with my patients, helping them to overcome or adapt, then regain their independence in their daily functioning.

The other consideration was that even though I tried to write this book informally—as if I were standing in front of you and your caregivers, attempting to present treatment strategies in written form—the book still shows the level of complexity that medical instructions do bear. I was inspired to use this as a relaxed teaching technique, hoping that I could pull it off. The reality is that anytime you attempt to write the instructions on how to perform a task, it's just easier to show them. Perhaps that is why YouTube is so popular. That is why my co-workers should always have gainful employment. It is for this reason that I hope my book can also assist or guide any new or currently working therapists in the treatment of their patients.

I hope this book helps to find you in good health. God bless.

VI

References

Cleveland Clinic. "Vital signs." Accessed March 17, 2020. *https://my.clevelandclinic.org/health/articles/10881-vital-signs.*

CWI Medical. "dressing stick-adaptive equipment." Accessed April 10, 2020. *https://www.cwimedical.com/sock-aid/dressing-aid-stick-dmi- das?*

FDA. "Dietary guidelines." Accessed June 20, 2020. *https://www.fda.gov/food/new-nutrition-facts-label/how-understand-and-use-nutrition-facts-label.*

Food and Nutrition Board, Institute of Medicine, National Academies. "Dietary Reference Intakes (DRIs): Recommended Dietary Allowances and Adequate Intakes, Total Water and Macronutrients." Accessed May 19, 2020. *https://www.ncbi.nlm.nih.gov/books/NBK56068/table/summarytables.t4/?report=objectonly.*

Health Products For You. "sock aid-adaptive equipment." Accessed April 10, 2020. *https://www.healthproductsforyou.*

com/p-sammons-preston-sock-and-stocking-aid-with-built-up-foam-handles.html?

Hopkins Medicine. "Hyperventilation-definition." Accessed April 4, 2020. *https://www.hopkinsmedicine.org/health/conditions-and-diseases/hyperventilation.*

Kansas. The Best of Kansas. Epic – EPC 461036 2, 1989, CD, Compilation, Reissue.

Olsen, M., *et al.* 2015. "Positive expiratory pressure – Common clinical applications and physiological effects." Journal of Respiratory Medicine, volume 109, (3):297-307. *https://doi.org/10.1016/j.rmed.2014.11.003.*

Piedmont healthcare. "Protein helps bond / carry o2 in blood to body" Accessed April 2, 2020. *https://www.piedmont.org/living-better/why-is-protein-important-in-your-diet.*

Ståhl, E., *et al.* "Health-related quality of life is related to COPD disease severity." *Health Qual Life Outcomes* (3):56. (2005). *https://doi.org/10.1186/1477-7525-3-56.*

USDA calories, MyPlate. "Learn your estimated calorie needs." Accessed June 20, 2020. *https://www.choosemyplate.gov/resources/MyPlatePlan.*

VII

Cheat Sheet: Breathing Exercises / Safety Considerations

Breathing Exercises

1. Puffy Cheeks Breathing-

- Breath in your nose, gently

- Exhale through mouth with puffy cheeks

- 2. Rib Cage Breathing-

- Breathe in nose while raising arms over your head

- Lower arms while blowing out using puffy cheeks

3. Diaphragm Breathing

- Poke your tummy out while gently inhaling

- Exhale and relax tummy while blowing out with puffy cheeks

- Do 3 sets of 5 repetitions for each above exercise

- Rest 15 seconds after each set of 5 repetitions

- Complete these 3 exercises 2-3 times a day, 5 times a week

Recommendation: Please see the preliminary instructions provided in this book prior to each of these breathing exercises. They will assist with understanding, safe setup, and effective performance.

SAFETY CONSIDERATIONS (page numbers are provided for a quick reference in book)

1. Assure that your physician is aware you are having shortness of breath with related fatigue, whether at rest or if it increases with activity. Page 13

2. General information: Always protect the patient with severe breathing conditions by using a clean, soft face mask. Ask that family or friends having cold or flu symptoms also wear a face mask when visiting.

3. Use puffy cheek breathing while breathing is heavy. The slight resistance created helps to get the bad air out. Page 40.

4. It is just as important to get the bad air out of your lungs (carbon dioxide) as it is to get the fresh air in (oxygen). Page 23.

5. A normal respiratory rate is 12-20 breaths per minute at rest. If it is greater than 24 breaths per minute at rest or less than 12 breaths per minute, notify your physician or seek medical attention immediately. Page 39.

6. To conserve your energy, use rest breaks before you need them. Page 67.

7. Breathe while exerting yourself. Avoid holding your breath when climbing stairs (Page 86), when putting socks on (Page 62), or during bowel movements (Page 89).

8. Planning ahead is the best way to conserve your energy. How do you pace yourself? Page 67.

9. Practice puffy cheeks breathing exercise in mirror to see what it looks like. Pages 31 and 38.

10. Quiz 1. While puffy cheek breathing, which should take longer: breathing in or out? Answer: breathing out. Page 41.

11. Quiz 2. While diaphragmatic breathing, which way does your tummy move when you inhale? Tummy moves inward or outward. Answer: outward. Page 51.

12. What is energy conservation, and how does it help breathing? Page 59.

13. Learn to breathe with your body movements. Page 58.

14. Ventilate the bathroom when bathing or showering. Page 96.

15. Use puffy cheek breathing to relax those muscles when anxious or during a stressful event (Page 81), when trying to sleep (Page 92), or when having pain (Page 81).

16. Eat smaller meals, or "mini meals," if your breathing becomes difficult after eating. Page 99.

17. Know your redline, a point in time in which an activity should stop to assure that you don't overdo it and can recover quickly. Page 83.

18. Learn how to take your respiratory rate to see how fast you are breathing. Page 39.

19. Positioning to support your breathing at rest and during exercises. Page 51.

20. Set yourself up to succeed. Be open and honest with yourself and ask for more help if needed. Page 55.

YouTube videos will be available to demonstrate breathing techniques instructed.

Made in the USA
Columbia, SC
22 November 2020

25213336R00065